HISTOLOGY

A TEXT AND PRACTICAL RECORD BOOK

HISTOLOGY
A TEXT AND PRACTICAL RECORD BOOK

Sangita Chauhan
Professor and Head
Department of Anatomy
Sawai Man Singh Medical College
Jaipur, Rajasthan, India

Seema Gupta
Professor
Department of Anatomy
Sawai Man Singh Medical College
Jaipur, Rajasthan, India

JAYPEE *The Health Sciences Publisher*
New Delhi | London | Philadelphia | Panama

Jaypee Brothers Medical Publishers (P) Ltd.

Headquarters
Jaypee Brothers Medical Publishers (P) Ltd.
4838/24, Ansari Road, Daryaganj
New Delhi 110 002, India
Phone: +91-11-43574357
Fax: +91-11-43574314
E-mail: jaypee@jaypeebrothers.com

Overseas Offices
J.P. Medical Ltd.
83, Victoria Street, London
SW1H 0HW (UK)
Phone: +44-20 3170 8910
Fax: +44 (0)20 3008 6180
E-mail: info@jpmedpub.com

Jaypee-Highlights Medical Publishers Inc.
City of Knowledge, Bld. 237, Clayton
Panama City, Panama
Phone: +1 507-301-0496
Fax: +1 507-301-0499
E-mail: cservice@jphmedical.com

Jaypee Medical Inc.
The Bourse
111, South Independence Mall East
Suite 835, Philadelphia, PA 19106, USA
Phone: +1 267-519-9789
E-mail: jpmed.us@gmail.com

Jaypee Brothers Medical Publishers (P) Ltd.
17/1-B, Babar Road, Block-B
Shaymali, Mohammadpur
Dhaka-1207, Bangladesh
Mobile: +08801912003485
E-mail: jaypeedhaka@gmail.com

Jaypee Brothers Medical Publishers (P) Ltd.
Bhotahity, Kathmandu, Nepal
Phone: +977-9741283608
E-mail: kathmandu@jaypeebrothers.com

Website: www.jaypeebrothers.com
Website: www.jaypeedigital.com

Inquiries for bulk sales may be solicited at: jaypee@jaypeebrothers.com

Histology: A Text and Practical Record Book

First Edition: **2015**

ISBN: 978-93-5152-654-4

Printed at Replika Press Pvt. Ltd.

Dedicated to

All our reverend teachers who taught us to question ourselves and to seek answers, and to all our students who are always curious.

Preface

Everything should be made as simple as possible, but no simpler.

—Einstein

Histology is a very specialized and vast field of medical science which involves the study of microscopic structures of the human body. Students find it very difficult to figure out and revise the entire histology course just before examinations, despite availability of several good textbooks on the subject. This problem has been further compounded ever since the duration of the course has been reduced to one year from one and a half years. It is an attempt to accustom the students to this vast study in a capsule form.

All important details have been covered sufficiently with labeled diagrams.

It is, however, emphasized that the book can be used in conjunction with a popular textbook that has stood the test of time.

It may be possible to improve the quality of the book. We would welcome critical appreciation from both students and teachers, as it will help in improving the subsequent edition of the book.

Sangita Chauhan
Seema Gupta

Contents

CHAPTER

1 Introduction

GENERAL INSTRUCTIONS

- The purpose of teaching histology provides a basis for understanding the internal structure of body tissues and organs.
- The students will study the stained section of tissues which are permanently preserved in the form of slides with the aid of an optical light microscope.
- Always wear apron in histology laboratory.
- Always bring *Histology: A Text and Record* in histology laboratory. It should be signed by the teacher-in-charge at the conclusion of each class.
- Bring liliac, violet, and black pencils and eraser.
- Handle the microscope and slides carefully and wipe clean after using it.
- Unless instructed, do not use high power.
- Not allowed to touch the slide or change the field of the slides which are kept for demonstration.
- Report any breakage to the laboratory staff immediately.

MICROSCOPE (FIGS 1.1 AND 1.2)

- The microscope is an instrument for the examination of cytological and histological specimens. There are many types of microscopes.
- Simple microscope is an ordinary magnifying glass having only one lens system and it gives less than 20 times magnification.
- Compound microscope has two lens systems. Objective lens and eyepiece lens. The image produced by objective lens is further magnified by the eyepiece lens.
- Magnification thus produced may range from 100 to 1500 times.
- In light microscopy, the day light or artificial light is used.
- Students will use compound light microscope.

The following are parts of compound microscope:

Mechanical	*Optical*
Body-tube, arm, foot	Eyepiece
Pillar, mechanical stage	*Objectives:* High power, low power, oil immersion
Coarse and fine adjustments	*Mirror:* Plane and concave surfaces on opposite sides
	Iris diaphragm
	Condenser

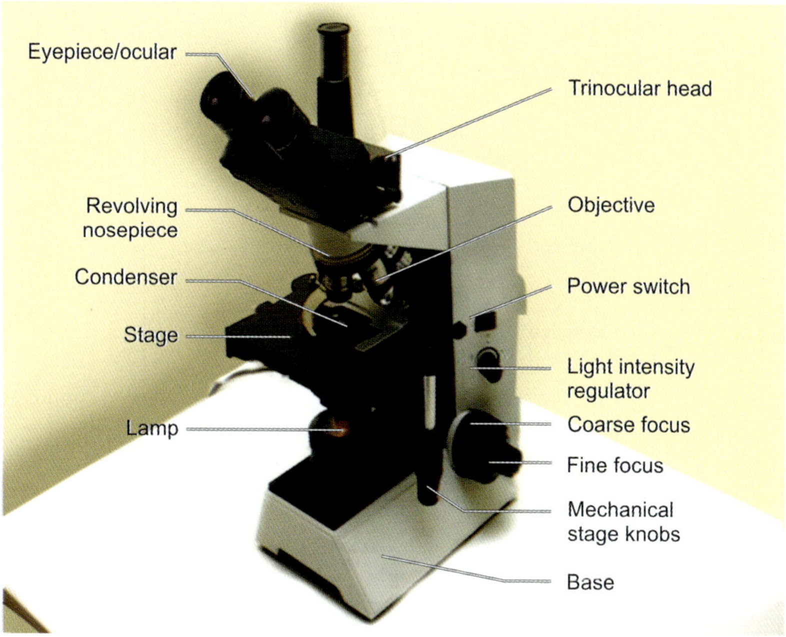

Fig. 1.1 Microscope

Blank space for sketch work by students

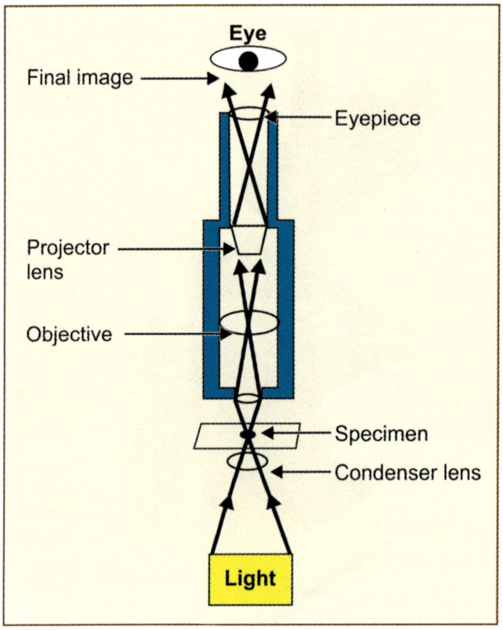

Fig. 1.2 Ray diagram

Blank space for sketch work by students

DARK GROUND MICROSCOPE

- In dark ground illumination, oblique light is thrown upon the object, which does not enter the objective, and the objects appear self-luminous on a dark background.
- In this method no direct rays of light from the condenser enter the objective and the objects are visible not because they are traversed by direct light entering the objective, but due to diffraction and reflection of indirect light rays into the objective.
- This method is more valuable for the examination of fresh specimens than for sections.

INTERFERENCE AND PHASE CONTRAST MICROSCOPY

- With an ordinary light microscope, it is very difficult to see unstained preparation of tissues.
- All cells and organisms, although appearing almost homogenous when examined unstained by ordinary light microscope, are composed of minute structures having slight difference in refractive index.
- The phase contrast microscope converts this slight difference of refractive index into changes of amplitude or brightness and produces an image that can be accurately focused and the same can easily, be seen or photographed.

FLUORESCENT MICROSCOPE

Tissues treated with a fluorescent dye when examined with ultraviolet light become luminous and are seen as bright objects against a dark field. This method is very widely used to study components of fungi, bacteria, etc.

ELECTRON MICROSCOPE

It is a refracting microscope in which instead of light rays, a stream of high velocity electrons is used. This is focused to form images of bodies far smaller than those perceptible by light. The image is photographed. The wavelength of these electrons is 1/1,00,000 of the wavelength of light.

- This microscope is constructed on the same optical principles as light microscope. Magnetic coils are used instead of lenses.
- Tissues are embedded in hard synthetic resin. Very thin sections of soft tissue are required. They are cut by glass or diamond knives.
- The sections are not stained.
- Magnifications to 2,00,000 times is produced.
- Resolution power is up to 1 nanometer units.

PARAFFIN SECTION STAINING: HEMATOXYLIN AND EOSIN METHOD

STAINING OF PARAFFIN SECTION

- Find the correct side of the slide on which the section lies.
- Heat gently the under surface of slide over a burner. Paraffin will be seen melting. Heating also coagulates the egg-albumin, dip in xylene two times for five minutes or keep it in the incubator overnight (37.3°C).
- Dip in xylene to dissolve the paraffin for 2–3 minutes.
- Hydrate the section gradually by dipping in descending grades of alcohol, i.e. absolute alcohol, then in 95%, 70% and 50%, 30%.
- Dip in distilled water.
- Stain with **Mayer's acidified hematoxylin** (Lillie's modification) for 5 minutes in **progressive staining method** and 7–10 minutes in regressive or retrogressive method. It stains the nuclei.
- Wash with tap water and see under the microscope to see the proper staining. If the section is over stained then do the next two steps.
- Dip in 0.025% HCl (or acidified alcohol) and remove the slide immediately. Acid removes the over staining.
- Wash the slide in running tap water for 5 minutes. It neutralizes the acid and turns the tissue blue in color. So known as **bluing process**.
- Wash with distilled water if necessary.
- Dehydrate the sections by dipping in ascending grades of alcohol, starting from 30%, 50%, 70%, 95% and absolute alcohol. This is done to preserve sections permanently.
- Counterstain with 1% eosin in 90% alcohol for ½–1 minute, until the cytoplasm and muscle cells if present take a deep pink stain. It stains the cytoplasm pink.
- Dry the slide by fanning in the air and dip in xylene, for clearing. Mount with digital picture exchange (DPX) or Canada balsam, which is soluble in xylene, at the same time refractive index is the same as that of glass. Put the cover slip. Do not use Canada balsam more than necessary.

  Clean the Canada balsam at the edge of the cover slip before putting the slide on the stage of microscope.

Results

- Nuclei—purplish blue (violet).
- Nucleolus—dark blue.
- Cytoplasm—pink.
- Other components varying according to tissues (Cartilage—pink or light blue).
- Collagen fibers and osteoid tissue—light pink.
- Muscle cells, thyroid colloids, thick elastic fibers—deep pink.

CHAPTER

2 General Histology

TISSUES

There are four basic types of tissues:
1. Epithelium
2. Connective tissue
3. Muscle
4. Nervous tissue.

MEMBRANOUS EPITHELIUM

- Epithelial cells are continuous sheets of cells comprising of one or more layers of cells.
- It covers the external surface of solid organs or lines the internal surface of hollow tubular structures and forms glands.
- Epithelial cells are adherent to each other by **cell junctions**.
- It is **avascular**, no blood vessels and lymphatics are found in the epithelium. Nutrition is by diffusion from supporting tissues.
- All epithelia are supported on basement membrane.
- All epithelial cells are **polarized** and have one free surface and a basal surface.
- Cells which lack free surface and are present as cell aggregates are classified as epithelioid tissues seen in certain endocrine glands.
- Epithelium has good **regenerative** capacity.
- When epithelium undergoes morphological and functional changes it is called **metaplasia**.
- Epithelium develops from all the three germ layers (**ectoderm**—epidermis, **mesoderm**—blood vessels and lymphatics, **endoderm**—gastrointestinal and respiratory).

Epithelia are present as single or multiple layers.

- **Simple Epithelium** single layer of cells of varying shapes.
  - *Simple squamous epithelium (Fig. 2.1)*
    - Flat cells, like scales of a fish.
    - Oval, flat nucleus in the center of the cell with very little cytoplasm. It is present in lung alveoli, Bowman's capsule and Henle's loop of renal tubules.
    - Lining of heart, blood vessels and lymphatics is called **endothelium**.
    - Lining of serous membranes of body cavities is called **mesothelium**.
    - It helps in rapid transport of substances, diffusion of gases and osmosis.

Keys for identification: Membranous epithelium (Squamous epithelium)

a. Flat, thin, scale like cell.
b. Oval, flat nucleus.
c. All cells rest on basement membrane.

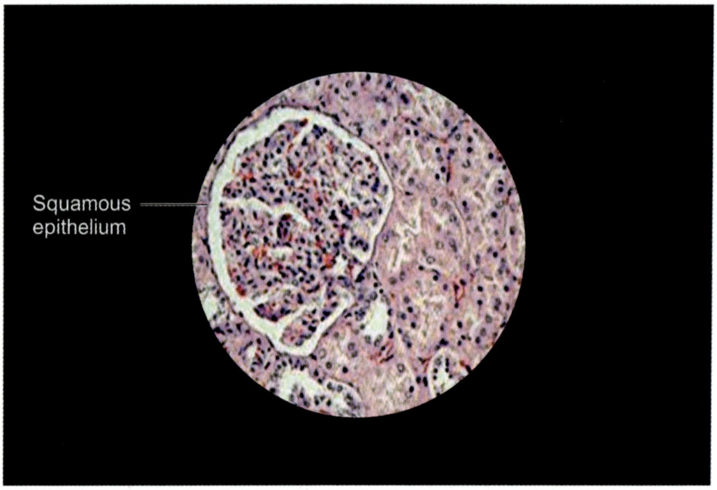

Fig. 2.1 Membranous epithelium (Squamous epithelium)

Blank space for sketch work by students

- *Simple cuboidal epithelium (Fig. 2.2)*
  - Single layer of cells.
  - Cells appear **square** with almost equal height, breadth and thickness.
  - Nucleus is round and centrally placed.

- Found in germinal epithelium of ovary, thyroid follicles, ducts of exocrine glands, proximal and distal tubules of kidney, pigment layer of retina.
- Concerned with secretion, absorption and excretion.

Keys for identification: Cuboidal epithelium

a. Single layer of square cells.
b. Nucleus is round and centrally placed.
c. All cells touch basement membrane.

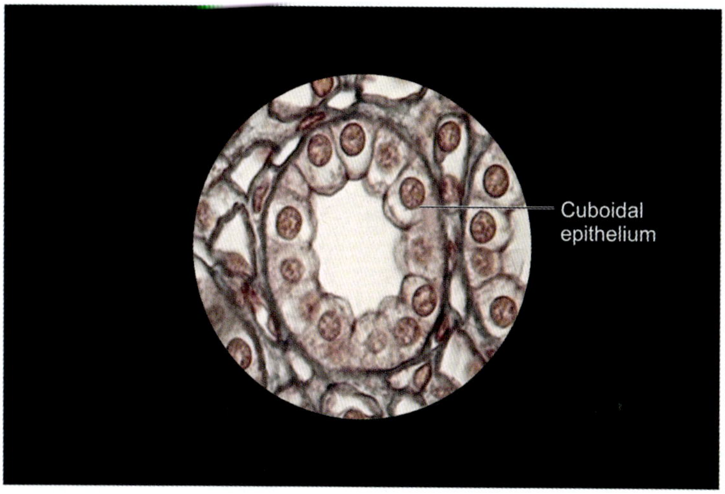

Fig. 2.2 Cuboidal epithelium

Blank space for sketch work by students

- *Simple columnar epithelium (Fig. 2.3)*
  - A single layer of cells which are **taller** than in width.
  - Nucleus is elongated and in the basal two-thirds of the cell.
  - Apical surface may be covered with cilia or microvilli.
  - Lines the stomach, intestines, rectum (GI tract), uterus, fallopian tubes, gallbladder and central canal of spinal cord. It is concerned with secretion, absorption and when ciliated, with propulsion of mucus.

Keys for identification: Columnar epithelium

a. Single layer of tall cells.
b. Elongated nucleus towards the base.
c. All cells rest on basement membrane.

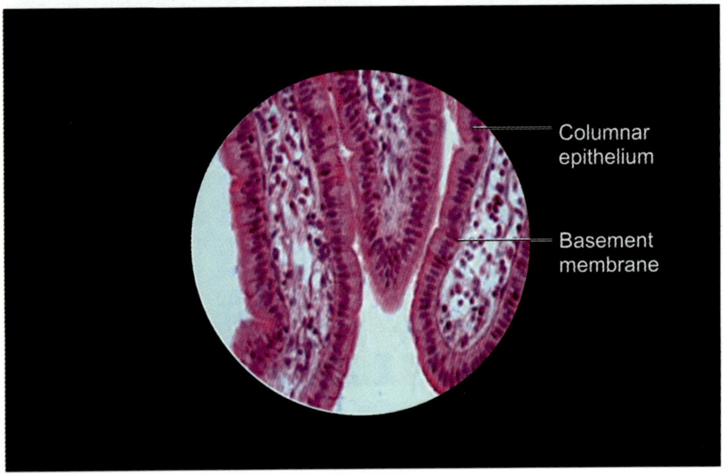

Fig. 2.3 Columnar epithelium

Blank space for sketch work by students

- *Pseudostratified columnar epithelium (Fig. 2.4)*
  - Variant of simple columnar epithelium.
  - Single layer of cells of variable shape and height with nuclei at different levels, hence **illusion of stratification**.
  - **All cells rest on basement membrane** but are of different height, hence all do not reach the apical surface.
  - May be ciliated or nonciliated.
  - May contain goblet cells.
  - Nonciliated epithelium is found in the large excretory ducts, auditory tube, male urethra, and male reproductive system (efferent ductules, epididymis, seminal vesicles and ductus deferens.
  - Ciliated epithelium lines upper respiratory tract.
  - Protects the underlying tissue.
  - Ciliary movement removes surface mucous and trapped foreign particles.

Keys for identification: Pseudostratified columnar epithelium

a. Single layer of different sized cells.
b. All cells rest on basement membrane.
c. Nuclei appear at different levels.

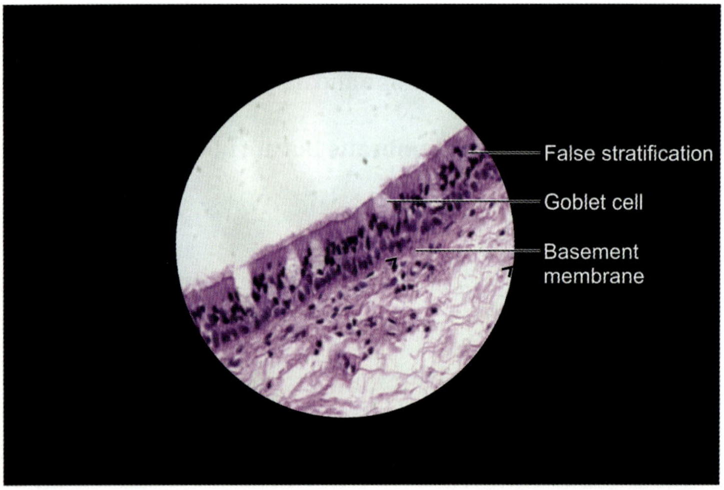

Fig. 2.4 Pseudostratified columnar epithelium

Blank space for sketch work by students

- **Stratified Epithelium** having two or more layers of cells.
  - *Stratified squamous epithelium: Keratinized (Fig. 2.5)*
    - Variable number of cell layers.
    - Surface cells are squamous, scale-like, horny, dead, enucleated and filled with the scleroprotein, **keratin**.
    - Deeper layers have polygonal cells in progressive stages of keratinization.
    - The basal layer has cuboidal to columnar cells and lies on basal lamina.
    - Superficial dead cells become hard and cornified where they are exposed to friction and wear and tear.
    - It is known as keratinized epithelium.
    - Keratinized epithelium is present in epidermis of skin.

Keys for identification: Stratified squamous epithelium: keratinized

a. Multilayered epithelium.
b. Surface layer is of squamous cells.
c. Most superficial layer is keratinized.

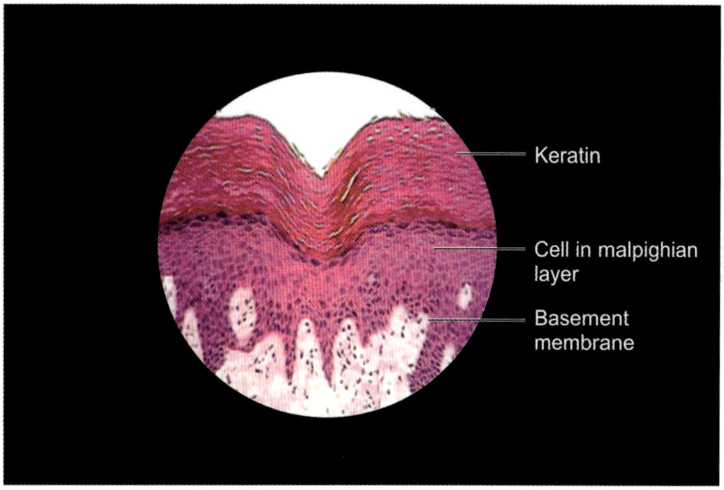

Fig. 2.5 Stratified squamous epithelium: keratinized

Blank space for sketch work by students

- *Stratified squamous epithelium: Nonkeratinized (Fig. 2.6)*
  - Nonkeratinized epithelium is found in similar but thinner surface.
  - Superficial cells are flat, nucleated and nonkeratinized.
  - Intermediate layers are polygonal cells.
  - The basal layer is cuboidal.

- It lines wet cavities, subject to abrasion (mouth, esophagus,, vagina, anal canal, vocal folds, cornea and tongue).
- It is less resistant to water loss than the keratinized type.

Keys for identification: Stratified squamous epithelium: nonkeratinized
a. Multilayered epithelium.
b. Superficial cells are squamous.
c. Surface layer is not covered by keratin.

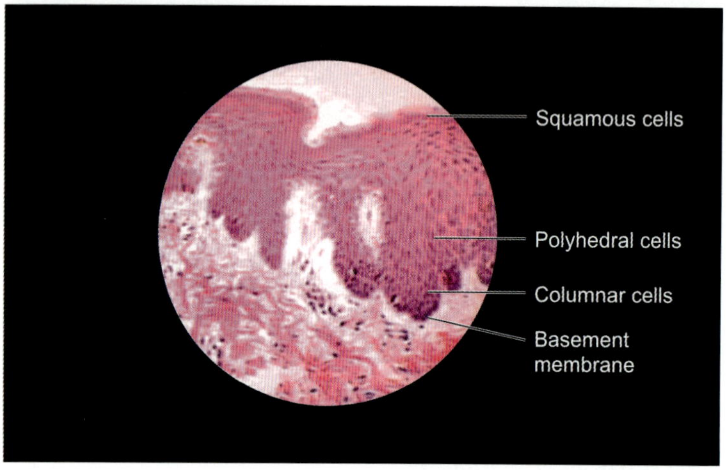

Fig. 2.6 Stratified squamous epithelium: nonkeratinized

Blank space for sketch work by students

- *Stratified cuboidal epithelium (Fig. 2.7)*
  - Multilayered, two to three layers seen.
  - Surface cells are cuboidal in shape.
  - Relatively rare and seen in ducts of salivary and sweat glands.
  - Concerned with limited absorption and protection.

Keys for identification: Stratified cuboidal epithelium

a. Cells in two to three layers.
b. Superficial layer is of cuboidal cells.
c. Basal layer may be cuboidal or columnar.

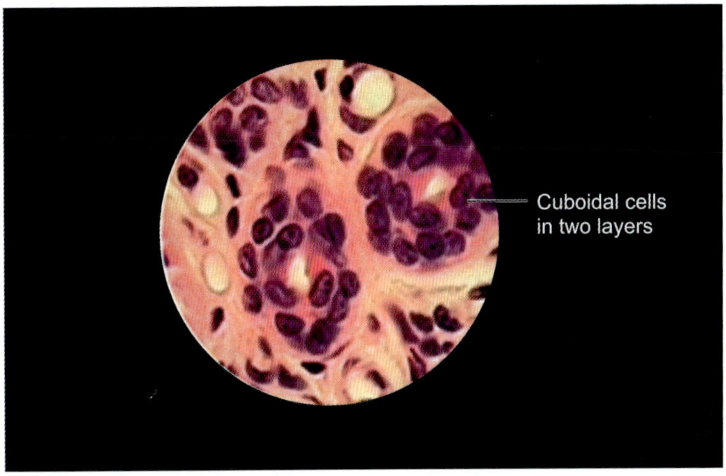

Fig. 2.7 Stratified cuboidal epithelium

Blank space for sketch work by students

- *Stratified columnar epithelium (Fig. 2.8)*
  - Multilayered, two to three layers.
  - Surface cells are columnar.
  - May be ciliated.
  - Lines the larger ducts of some glands, fornix of conjunctiva and urethra.
  - It sometimes, covers the respiratory surface of epiglottis.
  - Concerned with protection.

Keys for identification: Stratified columnar epithelium

a. Two to three layered cells.
b. Surface cells are columnar.
c. Basal layer may be cuboidal or columnar.

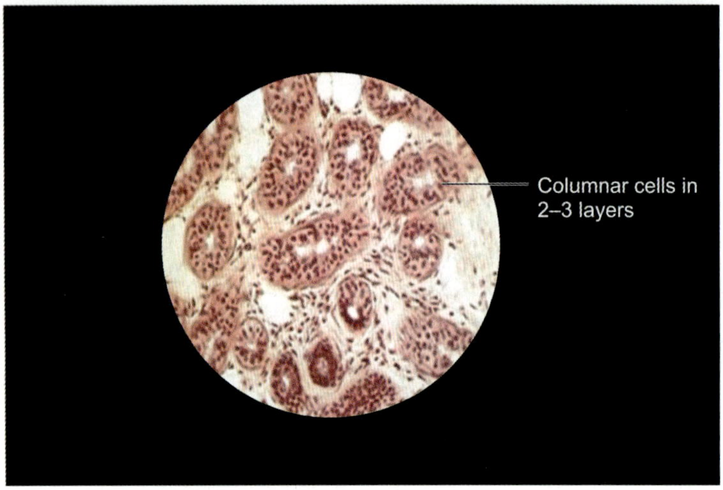

Fig. 2.8 Stratified columnar epithelium

Blank space for sketch work by students

TRANSITIONAL EPITHELIUM: UROTHELIUM (FIGS 2.9A AND B)

Multilayered

- Appearance varies during stretched and relaxed condition hence named **transitional**.
- When relaxed many layers of cells are seen but when stretched only two or three layers are seen.
- Deeper cells are cuboidal or polyhedral.
- Surface cells are large, dome or umbrella shaped and often binucleated.
- The luminal surface of the cells is scalloped, thick and darkly stained.
- It lines urinary passages hence called urothelium (renal calyces, pelvis, ureter, urinary bladder and proximal portion of urethra).

Keys for identification: Transitional epithelium

a. Multilayered epithelium lining the urinary tract (5–6 layers).
b. Cells lining the lumen are umbrella shaped.
c. Epithelium when stretched appears thinned out (2–3 layers).

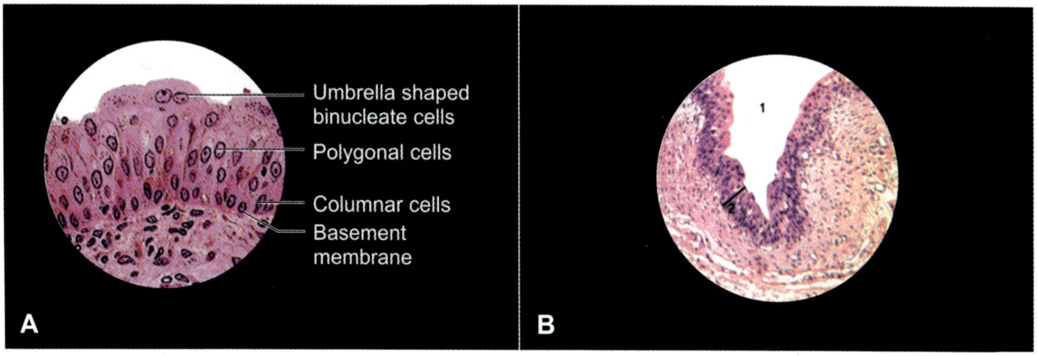

Figs 2.9A and B Transitional epithelium

Blank space for sketch work by students

SPECIALIZATIONS OF FREE SURFACE OF CELL

Microvilli

- Minute finger like projections of plasma membrane, 0.5–1 micron in length.
- Core contains many parallel actin microfilaments anchored in a dense mesh of filaments in the apical cytoplasm called terminal web.
- In the absorptive cells, apical surface is usually covered with microvilli which greatly increase the apical surface are for absorption.
- When regularly arranged—**striated** border, present in intestine.
- When irregularly arranged—**brush** border, seen in gallbladder and proximal tubules of kidney.

Functions

- Increased surface area by 15–30 times and hence increased absorption.
- Microvilli are nonmotile.
- In some microvilli, oscillatory contractile movements may be seen due to the presence of actin filaments.
- This helps in absorption.

Cilia

- Membrane covered cell surface extension about 10 microns in length
- Capable of rapid, regular and synchronous wavy movements.
- Short, fine hair like structures, arranged in rows on the apical cell surface.
- Shaft is covered by cell membrane.
- Core consists of central pair of microtubules with nine pairs of evenly spaced microtubules around them.
- At the base of cilia are basal bodies that are believed to have originated from centriole. Each basal body is similar in structure to centriole.
- Seen in respiratory tract (ciliated pseudostratified columnar epithelium) and oviducts (ciliated simple columnar epithelium) (Fig. 2.10).

Functions

Wave like movements of cilia helps to move the mucous in one direction (bronchus and tracheal epithelium). Responsible for the movement of ovum in oviduct.

Flagella

- A flagella is like a cilia but it is larger and longer and there are usually one or two per cell.
- Flagella occurs in tail of spermatozoa.

Stereocilia

- Nonmotile cilia are called stereocilia.
- Long cytoplasmic processes or microvilli.
- Structure resembles that of microvilli and therefore also called large microvilli.
- They lack in actin filaments in their core and are thus flexible.

Keys for identification: Ciliated columnar epithelium

a. Cilia on the apical part of the cell.
b. Columnar cells with oval nucleus towards the base of the cell.

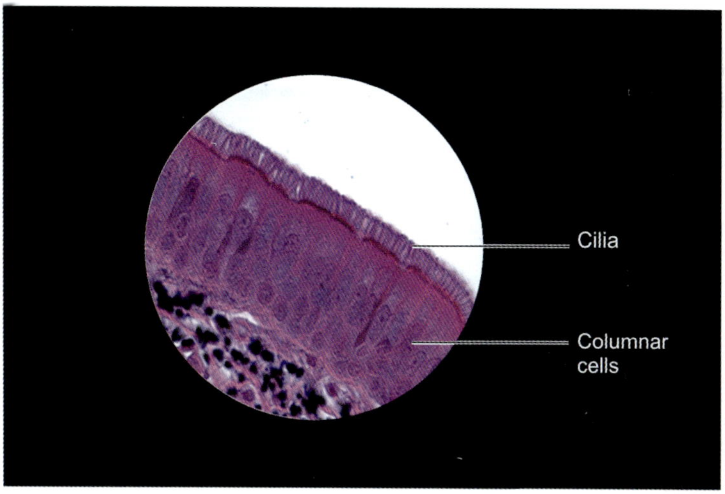

Fig. 2.10 Ciliated columnar epithelium

Blank space for sketch work by students

GLANDULAR EPITHELIUM

- Some epithelial cells have specialized function of secretion, such cells form the glands.
- These glands can be present as separate organs or as a part in the viscera.
- The epithelial cells grow inwards in underlying connective tissue, and secrete certain materials which can be enzymes, mucus, hormones or fat.
- Glands can be unicellular or multicellular.
- The proximal part of the invaginated epithelium forms the duct and it is in contact with the surface epithelium.
- The distal part forms the secretory unit.

TYPES OF GLANDS

- *Exocrine:* Here they pour their secretions on the surface by a duct, e.g. salivary glands.
- *Endocrine:* Some glands lose their surface contact and pour their secretions directly in the blood, e.g. thyroid, ovary, testis, etc.
- *Paracrine:* Secretes their substance locally which affects the surrounding cells, e.g. entero-endocrine cells of GIT.

Based on Number of Cells

Unicellular: Single cell, e.g. goblet cell in GIT, respiratory system.

Multicellular: All the other glands.

Based on Duct System

Simple: Single duct which does not branch.

Compound: Branching duct system.

Based on Shape of Secretory Unit

Tubular: Elongated tubular cells.

Alveolar/Acinar: Grapelike.

Tubuloalveolar: Mixed.

Further Subclassification

- *Simple tubular:* Crypts of Liberkuhn.
- *Simple coiled tubular:* Sweat glands.
- *Simple branched tubular:* Fundic and uterine glands.
- *Simple acinar:* Mucus glands of penile urethra.
- *Simple branched acinar:* Sebaceous gland and tarsal glands.

- *Compound tubular:* Brunner's glands of duodenum.
- *Compound acinar:* Parotid, mammary gland and exocrine of pancreas.
- *Compound tubuloalveolar:* Submandibular gland.

Based on Mode of Secretion

- *Merocrine:* Cells release their contents by exocytosis, e.g. pancreas and parotid.
- *Apocrine:* Apical part of cytoplasm of secretory cell is lost in the process of secretion lipids of mammary gland.
- *Holocrine:* Whole cell gets disintegrated to discharge the secretion, e.g. sebaceous gland.
- *Cytocrine/cytogenic gland:* Glands secrete cells instead of chemical substances, e.g. testes release sperms, ovary—ova, lymph nodes—lymphocytes.

Based on Nature of Secretion

- *Serous (Fig. 2.11):* Cells are small sized, pyramidal shaped.
  - Nucleus is round, darkly stained, in the center.
  - Lumen is small or obliterated.
  - Apical portion is filled with pinkish granules.
  - Basal portion shows basophilia.
  - Present in parotid gland and exocrine pancreas.

Keys for identification: Glandular epithelium (Serous acini)

a. Pyramidal shaped cells with round nucleus.
b. Lumen is small or obliterated.
c. Apical portion filled with granules.

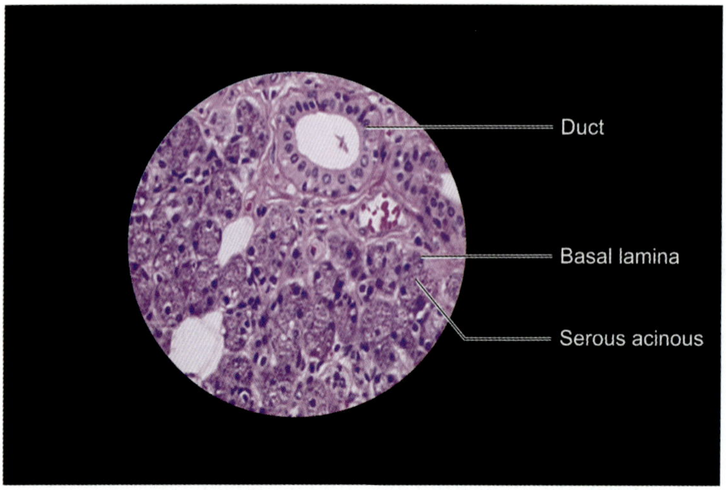

Fig. 2.11 Glandular epithelium (Serous acini)

Blank space for sketch work by students

- *Mucous (Fig. 2.12):* Cells are large in size, columnar to pyramidal.
  - Lumen is large.
  - Lightly stained cells.
  - Flat nucleus is towards the base of the cells.
  - Thick mucous secretion.
  - Apical portion of cell contains mucin granules which do not take H and E stain.
  - Present in sublingual gland.

Keys for identification: Mucous acini

a. Cells are large, columnar to pyramidal.
b. Flat nucleus towards base.
c. Cells filled with mucin.

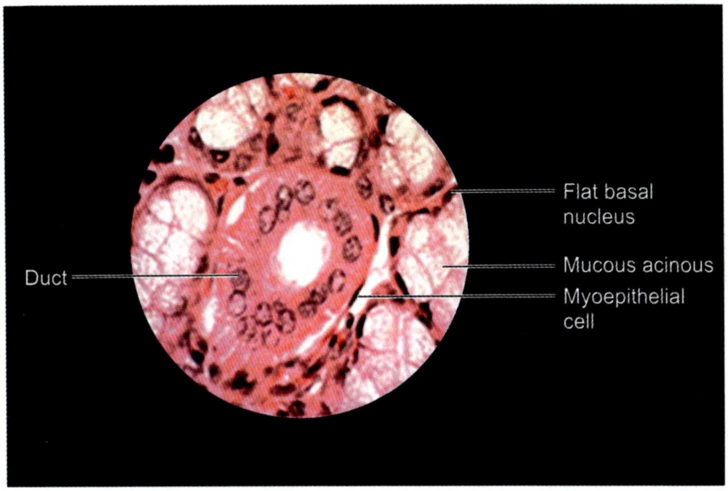

Fig. 2.12 Mucous acini

Blank space for sketch work by students

- *Mixed (Fig. 2.13):* Both serous and mucous fluid, seen in submandibular gland.
  - The mucous acini are capped with half moon shaped serous acinus called demilunes.
  - Both drain into the same acinus.

Keys for identification: Mixed acini

a. Mixed acini, both serous and mucous are seen.
b. Serous demilunes are seen.
c. Mucous acini are lightly stained.

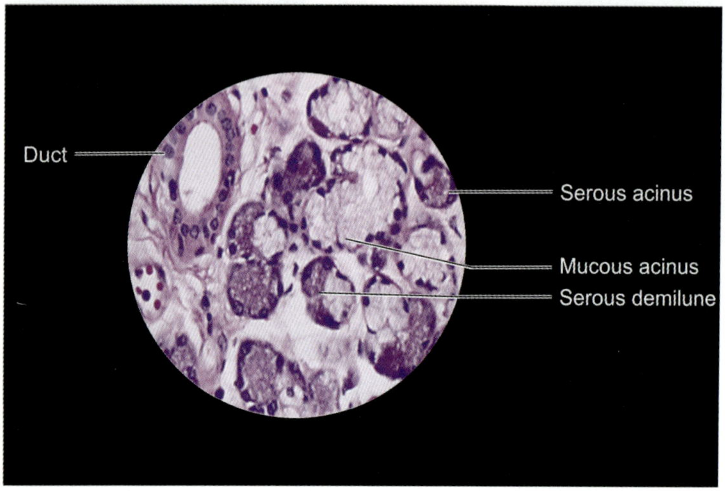

Fig. 2.13 Mixed acini

Blank space for sketch work by students

CONNECTIVE TISSUE

- It is one of the basic tissues which give structural and metabolic support to other tissues and organs throughout the body.
- Its two main components are **cells** and **extracellular matrix**. The cells synthesize the matrix.
- The **extracellular matrix** determines the physical properties of each type of supporting tissue.
- It consists of **fibers** and **ground substance**.
- Hence, connective tissue has cells, fibers and ground substance.

Functions: Important in binding or packing, support, compartmentalization and providing strength, storage, defence, transport and repair.

CELLS OF CONNECTIVE TISSUE

Resident cells or fixed cells: They are native to the tissue.

Mesenchymal cells: They are loose network of stellate cells which are precursors of most of the connective tissue.

Fibroblasts: They are most common cell seen, flat, fusiform in shape with slender processes.
- They synthesize extracellular matrix with fibers and ground substance.
- The old inactive fibroblasts are called **fibrocytes**.
- Fibroblasts with contractile properties are known as **myofibroblasts**. They are seen in sites of wound healing.

Adipocytes (fat cells): They synthesize and store fat.
- They are spherical in shape, **signet ring** appearance, due to flat nucleus displaced on one side and whole cell is filled with lipid.

Pigment cells (Melanocytes): They are star shaped cells with many processes.
- They produce melanin found in skin and iris.

Fixed macrophages (Histiocytes): They are irregular in shape with many filopodial processes.
- They have eccentrically placed nucleus and are derived from blood monocytes.
- Play important role in defence of the body by phagocytosis of foreign particles.

Plasma cells: They are derived from B lymphocytes.
- They have eccentric round nucleus with clumps of chromatin giving **cartwheel** appearance.
- They produce antibodies against antigen and involved in defence of body.

Mast cells: They are small, round or fusiform in shape.
- Nucleus is round and central and cytoplasm contains granules which gives metachromatic appearance.
- It releases histamine.
- They are found along small blood vessels.

Leukocytes: Nucleated white blood cells may migrate to connective tissue from blood vessels through a process of **diapedesis**.

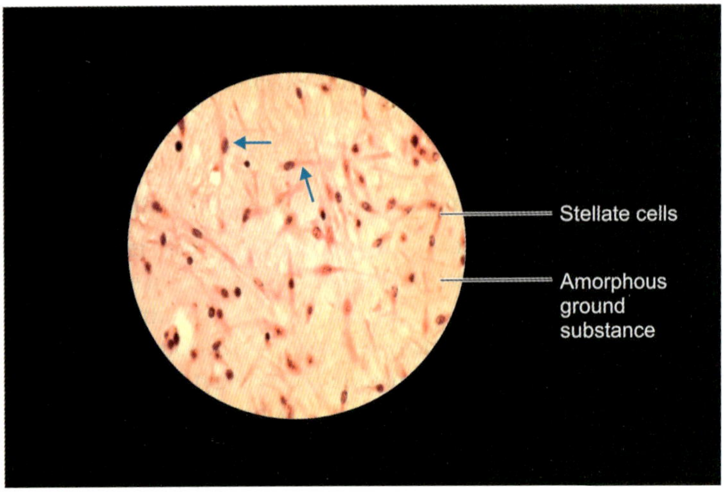

Fig. 2.14 Connective tissue (Mucoid connective tissue)

Blank space for sketch work by students

LOOSE AREOLAR CONNECTIVE TISSUE (FIG. 2.15)

- Most widely spread connective tissue.
- It has loose network of collagen, elastic and reticular fibers with tissue cells.
- Ground substance has hyaluronic acid and chondroitin sulphate.
- For example, lamina propria, superficial fascia, around blood vessels, nerves and muscles.
- It conveys nutrients and oxygen to the tissue.

Keys for identification: Loose areolar connective tissue

a. Long wavy collagen fibers.
b. Short branching elastic fibers.
c. Different types of connective tissue cells.

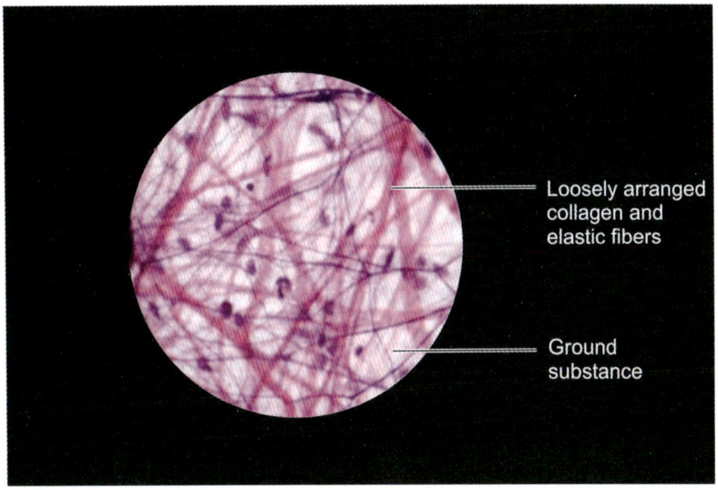

Fig. 2.15 Loose areolar connective tissue

Blank space for sketch work by students

DENSE CONNECTIVE TISSUE

Dense Irregular Connective Tissue (Fig. 2.16)

- It has haphazard bundles of type I collagen.
- In ground substance fibers form compact network with little spaces occupied by cells.
- For example, dermis, dura mater, epimysium, epineurium, pericardium, periosteum, tunica albuginea of testis, sclera, submucosa of GIT, capsule of various organs.

Keys for identification: Dense irregular connective tissue

a. Matrix is relatively acellular.
b. It contains high proportion of collagen bundles in all directions.
c. Few flattened fibroblasts are seen.

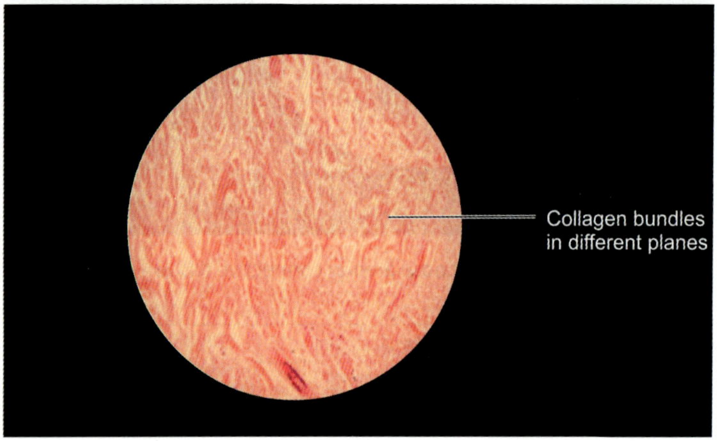

Fig. 2.16 Dense irregular connective tissue

Blank space for sketch work by students

Dense Regular Connective Tissue (Fig. 2.17)

- It consists of tightly packed bundles of collagen type I with very little space.
- For example, tendons, aponeuroses, ligaments, periosteum, deep fascia, and perichondrium

Keys for identification: Dense regular connective tissue longitudinal section (LS) of a tendon

a. Highly fibrous tissue where fibers are regularly oriented.
b. Direction of fibers is related to stress.
c. The trapped fibroblasts become compressed and appear stellate shaped.

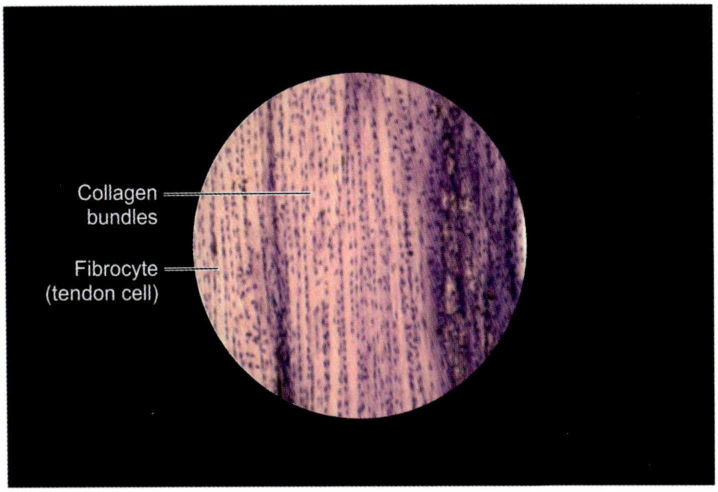

Fig. 2.17 Dense regular connective tissue longitudinal section (LS) of a tendon

Blank space for sketch work by students

RETICULAR TISSUE (FIG. 2.18)

- Delicate network of reticular fibers form **structural support** and framework.
- Poorly stained with H and E stain, silver stains are used, appear black.
- For example, bone marrow, lymph node, spleen, liver, around smooth muscle and reticular lamina.

Keys for identification: Reticular connective tissue

a. Fine branching fibers form the supporting framework of many organs.
b. They are type III collagen and stain intensely with silver salts.

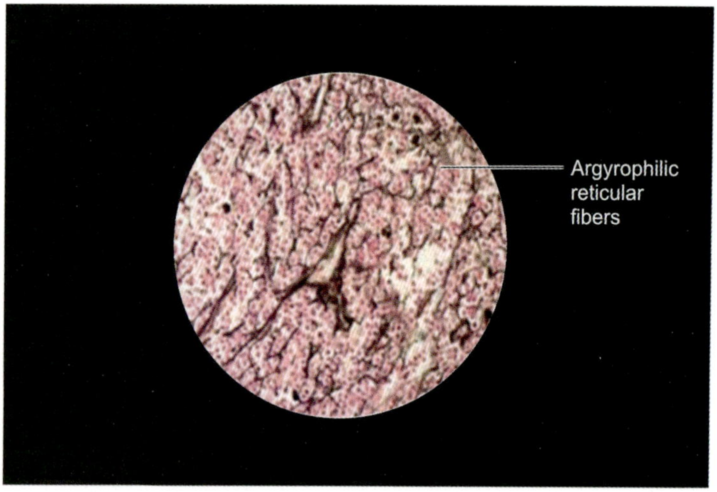

Fig. 2.18 Reticular connective tissue

Blank space for sketch work by students

ELASTIC TISSUE (FIG. 2.19)

- The insoluble elastin protein forms elastic fibers.
- Elastic fibers predominantly present, appear as **wavy** parallel bundles.
- They are separated by loose collagenous tissue.
- Provides flexibility and elasticity to the tissue.
- For example, wall of large arteries, ligamentum nuchae, ligamentum flava, vocal cords, fascia of anterior abdominal wall.

Keys for identification: Elastic connective tissue longitudinal section (LS)

a. Elastic fibers are wavy in appearance.
b. They accommodate changes in shape and volume.
c. Need special stain like orcein.

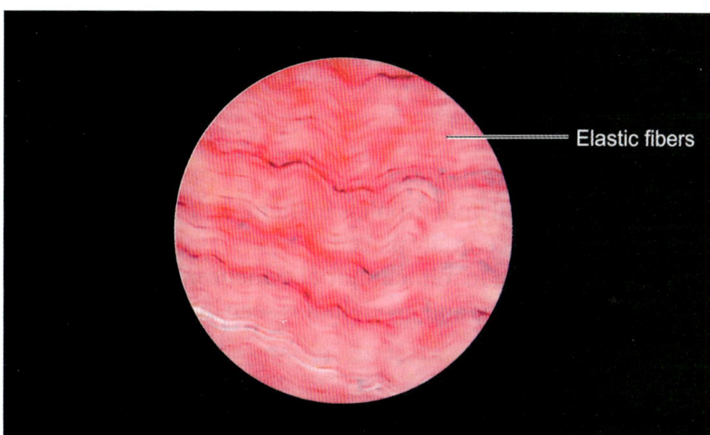

Fig. 2.19 Elastic connective tissue longitudinal section (LS)

Blank space for sketch work by students

ADIPOSE TISSUE (FIG. 2.20)

- In this special connective tissue, adipocytes store intracellular fat in form of lipid droplets.
- It constitutes 15–20% of body weight in men and 20–25% in women.
- Clusters of adipocytes are divided into lobules and lobes by fibrous septae.

White Adipose Tissue

- Unilocular adipose tissue.
- Found just beneath the skin, omentum, mesentry, around kidneys, orbits, joints and palms and soles.
- A mature adipocyte has lipid droplets occupying almost the whole cell, displacing the nucleus and cytoplasm to the periphery giving **"signet ring"** appearance.
- It is vascularized.
- It has a role in energy storage, endocrine function, insulation and cushion against mechanical shock.
- It is deficient in eyelids, scrotum, penis, external ear, scalp, etc.

Brown Adipose Tissue

- It is multilocular type of adipose tissue.
- Adipocytes have multiple small lipid droplets in them.
- Cells are smaller and nucleus centrally placed.
- It is reddish brown in color due to mitochondrial cytochrome and rich blood supply.
- It is most prominent in newborns and in adults it is seen in axilla, thyroid gland, renal hilus and near carotid artery.

Keys for identification: Adipose tissue

a. Rounded or oval or polygonal cells.
b. Lobules with interlobular septum.
c. Signet ring appearance.

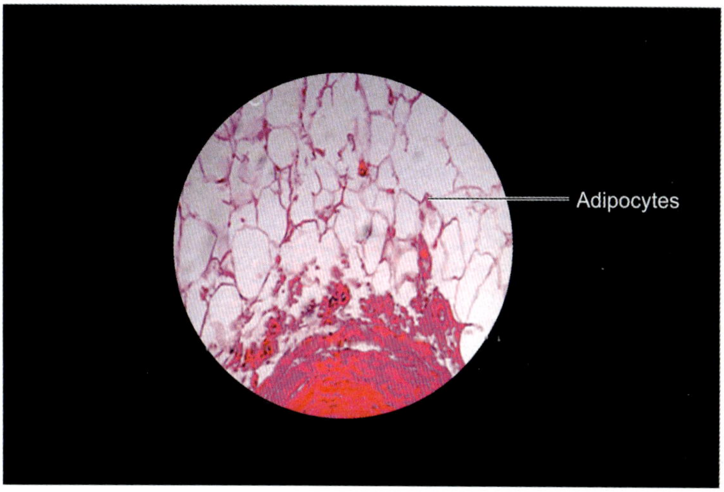

Fig. 2.20 Adipose tissue

Blank space for sketch work by students

CARTILAGE

- Cartilage is special connective tissue formed by chondroblasts.
- It is **firm and resilient**.
- It is composed of chondrocytes and glycosaminoglycans with collagen fibers.
- It is avascular and enveloped by perichondrium which contains vascular supply and fibroblastic stem cells.

  There are three types of cartilage:

HYALINE CARTILAGE (HYALOS—GLASS) (FIG. 2.21)

- Cartilage cells occur in encapsulated isogenous groups forming cell nests.
- Cells are present in lacunae in groups of 2, 4, 6, etc.
- Ground substance appears homogeneous and takes light blue stain (glassy appearance).
- It contains fine collagen fibers type III whose refractive index is close to ground substance and hence difficult to delineate.
- Basophilic matrix has chondroitin and keratan sulphate.
- Matrix near the cell nests is more basophilic and is known as territorial matrix and matrix between the cell nests is known as inter-territorial cell matrix.
- Perichondrium covers hyaline cartilage except articular cartilage.
- It has two layers, outer fibrous and inner cellular layer forming chondroblasts.
- Development and growth occurs both interstitial and appositional type.
- It is found in fetal skeleton, ends of long bones, epiphyseal and articular cartilage, nose, costal cartilage, trachea, bronchi, thyroid, cricoid and basal parts of arytenoid cartilage.

Keys for identification: Cartilage (Hyaline cartilage)

a. Groups of encapsulated cells (Chondrocytes forming cell nests).
b. Homogenous ground substance or matrix (glass like).
c. Outermost perichondrium.

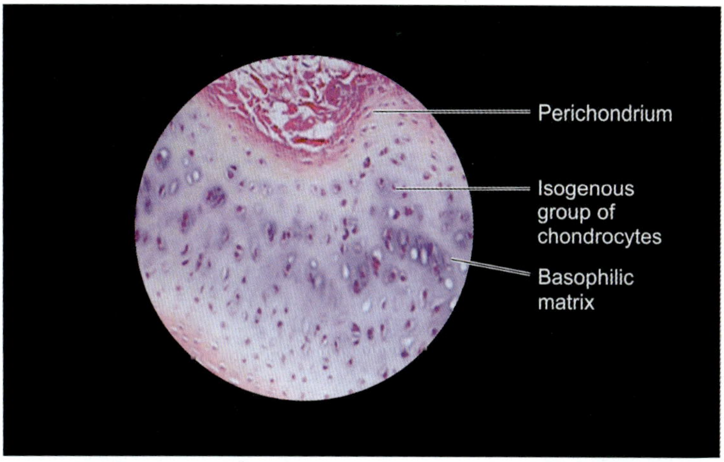

Fig. 2.21 Cartilage (Hyaline cartilage)

Blank space for sketch work by students

ELASTIC CARTILAGE (FIG. 2.22)

- The structure is same as hyaline cartilage.
- The chondrocytes are larger and occur **singly**.
- The matrix contains elastic fibers which are not visible because they do not take H and E stain. They are visualized by special stain, like orcein.
- It has perichondrium and similar growth pattern like hyaline cartilage.
- It occurs in external ear, auditory tube and canal, epiglottis, corniculate and cuneiform cartilages of larynx.

Keys for identification: Elastic cartilage

a. Matrix have dense network of elastic fibers.
b. Scattered large cartilage cells.
c. Perichondrium present.

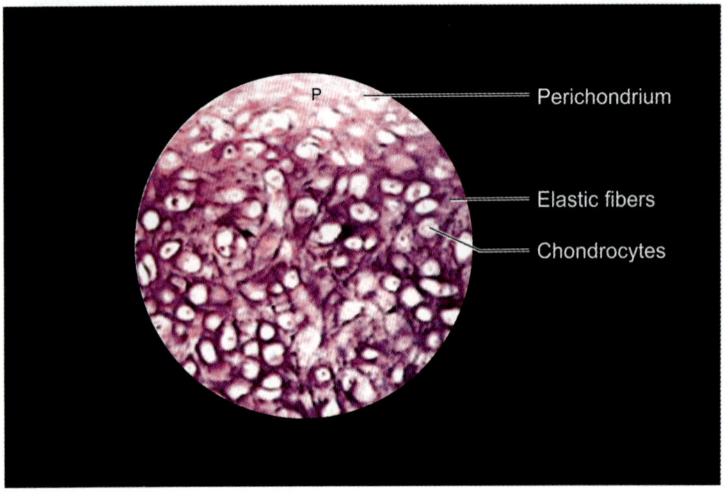

Fig. 2.22 Elastic cartilage

Blank space for sketch work by students

FIBROCARTILAGE (FIG. 2.23)

- The chondrocytes are small and fewer in number, and lie in a **row**.
- Intercellular matrix is thick and contains abundant irregular bundles of collagen type I.
- Perichondrium is **absent**.
- It is seen in intervertebral disc, pubic symphysis, articular disc of joints, menisci, acetabular labrum and sites of insertion of tendons in bone.

Keys for identification: Fibrocartilage

a. Rounded few cartilage cells (chondrocytes) are arranged in rows.
b. Matrix has abundance of thick bundles of collagen fibers
c. Absence of perichondrium.

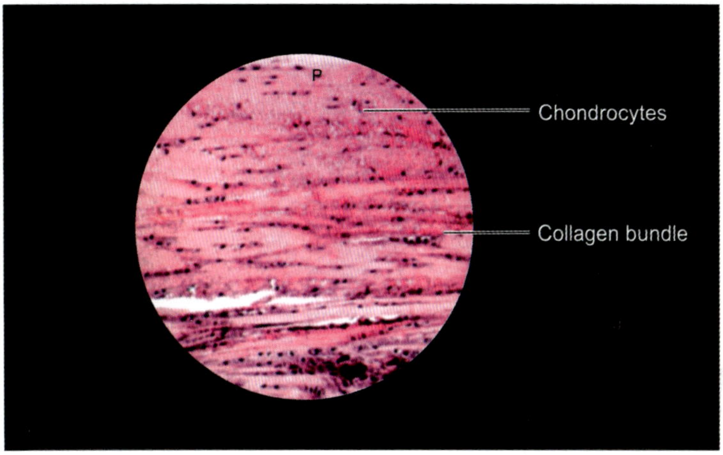

Fig. 2.23 Fibrocartilage

Blank space for sketch work by students

BONE TISSUE

- It is **dynamic** specialized type of connective tissue.
- It is composed of **cells** and **extracellular matrix** called osteoid.
- It becomes mineralized by calcium hydroxyapatite crystals giving rigidity and strength.

CELLS

- *Osteoprogenitor cells*—these are spindle shaped stem cells found in endosteum and periosteum.
- *Osteoblasts*—these are bone forming cells which are cuboidal with round nucleus and basophilic cytoplasm. They synthesize matrix.
- *Osteocytes*—these are differentiated bone cells found in small spaces in bony matrix called lacunae.

  Thin cytoplasmic processes called filopodia radiate from the cell body and extend in small canaliculi of the lacunae.
- *Osteoclasts*—bone resorbing cells.
  - These are large multinucleate cells lying in depressions resorbed from the bone called **Howships** lacunae.
  - It has ruffled border facing the bone which secretes organic acids.
  - Parathyroid hormone stimulates osteoclastic activity and releases calcium from the bone, whereas calcitonin inhibits osteoclastic activity.

Bone matrix: Newly formed matrix is **osteoid** which forms 25% of bone weight.
- It contains organic components, fibers and ground substance.
- Fibers are mainly type I collagen.
- Glycosaminoglycans are chondroitin sulphate and keratan sulphate. The glycoproteins are osteonectin, osteocalcin and osteopontin.
- Inorganic components are crystals of hydroxyapatite of calcium, phosphate along with potassium, magnesium bombesin and citrate.

WOVEN (SPONGY BONE) (FIG. 2.24)

- Found in epiphysis, flat bones, irregular bones, all short bones, thin rim around cavity of diaphysis of long bones and healing bones.
- It has meshwork of bony spicules or trabeculae which anastomose with each other.
- There are small numerous spaces that are filled with bone marrow.

Keys for identification: Bone (Woven bone)
a. Bony trabeculae seen.
b. Spaces filled with bone marrow.
c. Osteoblasts and osteocytes seen.

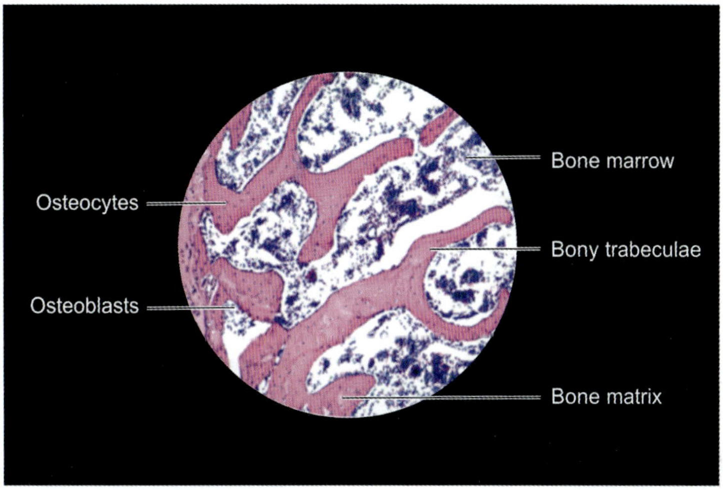

Fig. 2.24 Bone (Woven bone)

Blank space for sketch work by students

COMPACT (LAMELLAR BONE) (FIGS 2.25 AND 2.26)

- It is present in diaphysis of long bone and thin layer on external surface of all the other bones.
- Outer and inner surface is covered with periosteum and endosteum respectively.
- Lamellae are seen in three different patterns.

Haversian system or **osteon,** consists of concentric lamellae around a central Haversian canal which contains loose connective tissue, capillaries, nerves and lymphatics.

Between the lamellae there are oval spaces lacunae with osteocytes.

Volkmann's canal are horizontal or obliquely placed canals which communicate the two Haversian canals or a canal with surface periosteum for blood vessels and nerves.

Cement line is a zone of mineralized matrix with collagen surrounding each osteon.

Keys for identification: Compact bone transverse section (TS)

a. Presence of osteons (Haversian system).
b. Haversian canal at the center containing blood vessels.
c. Presence of lamellae, lacunae, canaliculi and osteocytes.

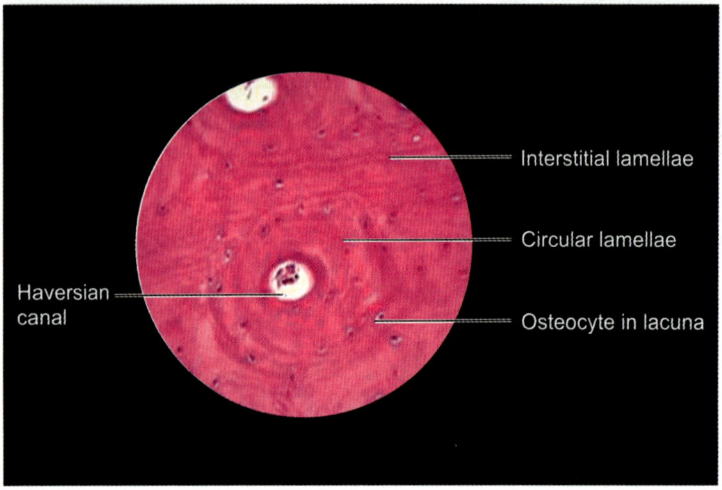

Fig. 2.25 Compact bone transverse section (TS)

Blank space for sketch work by students

Keys for identification: Bone longitudinal section (LS)

a. Longitudinal sections of Haversian canals.
b. Horizontal sections of Volkmann's canal.
c. Different types of lamellae.

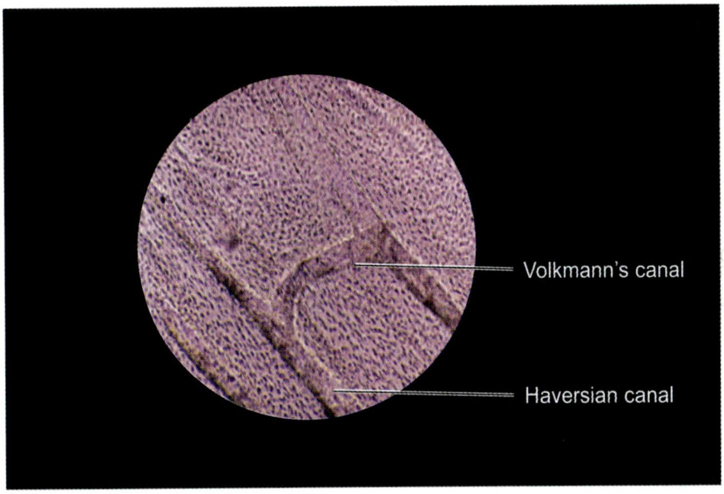

Fig. 2.26 Bone longitudinal section (LS)

Blank space for sketch work by students

PERIOSTEUM

- It is the external lining of the bones.
- It has outer fibrous and inner cellular layer which is osteogenic.
- Blood vessels of periosteum supply nutrition to the developing bone.
- **Sharpey's fibers** are collagenous or tendinous fibers which pass through periosteum and continue into the outer layers of the bone.

ENDOSTEUM

- Inner lining of the bone that faces the marrow cavity.
- It consists of resting cells which are flat and squamous type.

ENDOCHONDRAL OSSIFICATION (DEVELOPING BONE) (FIG. 2.27)

- Here cartilage is replaced by bone.
- Initially **mesenchymal model** is formed by the mesenchymal cells.
- The cells differentiate into chondroblasts, forming **cartilage hyaline model**.

As the bone is formed many stages of development are identified.

Zone of reserve cartilage—typical hyaline cartilage is seen.

Zone of proliferation—the chondrocytes proliferate forming longitudinal columns separated by strongly stained matrix.

Zone of cartilage degeneration—cartilage cells increase in size and the intercellular matrix becomes calcified, which cannot transfer nutrition by diffusion.

Zone of new bone formation by osteogenic, vascular bud.

Zone of resorption—osteoclasts resorb the destroyed bone.

Keys for identification: Endochondral ossification (Developing bone)

a. Zone of hyaline cartilage.
b. Long columns of chondrocytes.
c. Zone of cartilage degeneration and bone formation.

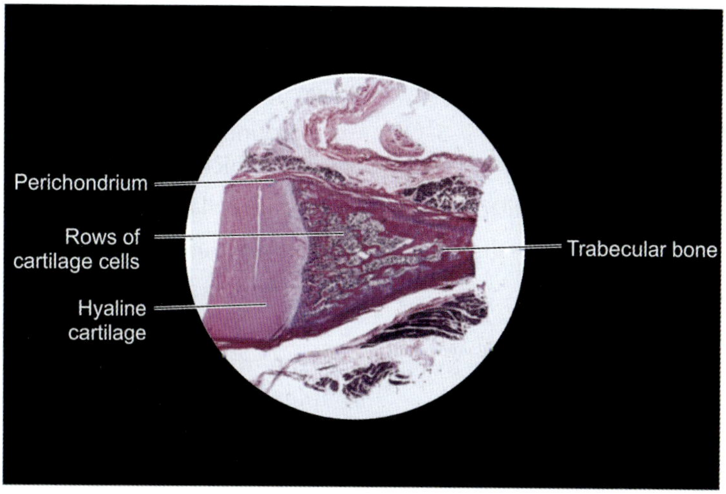

Fig. 2.27 Endochondral ossification (Developing bone)

Blank space for sketch work by students

Differences between Cartilage and Bone

Cartilage	*Bone*
It is firm but flexible tissue	The ground substance is made up of proteoglycans which are in low concentration
Fibers vary as per the type of cartilage	Fibers are collagenous
Matrix does not contain mineral salts	Mineral salts are deposited in matrix
Lacunae contain chondrocytes	Lacunae contain osteocytes with the protoplasmic processes
Cells receive nutrients by diffusion through matrix	As the matrix is mineralized diffusion of nutrients is not possible. Hence, canaliculi serve as means for passage of nutrients.
Collagen fibers are not organized to form lamellae	Collagen fibers are organized in lamellae
Cartilage grows by interstitial and appositional growth	Bone grows only by appositional growth

MUSCLE

- These are specialized cells which generate **motile forces** by interaction of proteins actin and myosin.
- Four main groups of contractile cells are:
  1. All muscle cells
  2. Myoepithelial cells
  3. Myofibroblasts
  4. Pericytes.
- Muscle cells comprise striated, cardiac and smooth muscles.
- Cells are longer than their breadth therefore called muscle fibers.

SKELETAL MUSCLE/STRIATED/VOLUNTARY (FIGS 2.28 AND 2.29)

- All are attached to the bone and derived from mesenchyme of mesoderm.
- The skeletal muscle cell components are named as **sarcolemma** (cell membrane), sarcoplasm (cytoplasm) and **sarcoplasmic reticulum** (endoplasmic reticulum).
- Each cell is a long cylindrical structure with 50–60 mm diameter and length from 100 mm to 35 cm depending on location.
- The muscle fiber is unbranched, cylindrical cell with numerous flattened nuclei just beneath the sarcolemma.
- Every fiber is surrounded by external lamina and has **resident satellite cells** which can form new muscle cells after damage.
- Contractile elements are **myofibrils** which are 1–24 mm in diameter.
- They are overlapping thick and thin filaments arranged in repeating assemblies.
- There are alternate zones of thick and thin filaments in a striated muscle.
- Muscle fiber also contains Golgi bodies, mitochondria, endoplasmic reticulum and myoglobin.
- In light microscope alternate light and dark bands are seen.
- *Dark:* A (Anisotropic) band
- *Light:* I (Isotropic) band.
- *Z line:* Dark transverse line in the middle of I band.
- *H band:* Light transverse line in the middle of A band.
- *M line:* Dark line in middle of H band.
- *Sarcomere* is between two Z lines.
- Individual muscle fibers are grouped into bundles called fasciculi with delicate supporting tissue called endomysium.
- Each fascicle is surrounded by **perimysium**.
- Whole muscle is surrounded by connective tissue sheath called **epimysium** through which large blood vessels and nerves enter.

- In transverse section fibers appear polyhedral with flattening of adjacent cells. Nuclei are present at periphery and small capillaries are seen between the spaces. Striations are not seen in cross-sections.

Keys for identification: Muscular tissue (Skeletal muscle LS)

a. Prominent transverse striations (alternate dark and light bands).
b. Peripherally situated flattened multiple nuclei.
c. Long cylindrical muscle cells.

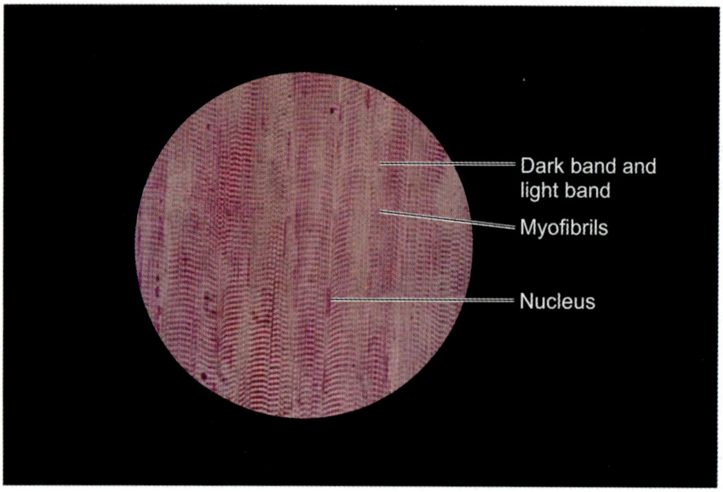

Fig. 2.28 Muscular tissue (Skeletal muscle LS)

Blank space for sketch work by students

Keys for identification: Skeletal muscle (TS)

a. Peripherally nucleated muscle bundles or fascicles.
b. Perimysium around the muscle fascicles.
c. Epimysium covering the whole muscle tissues.

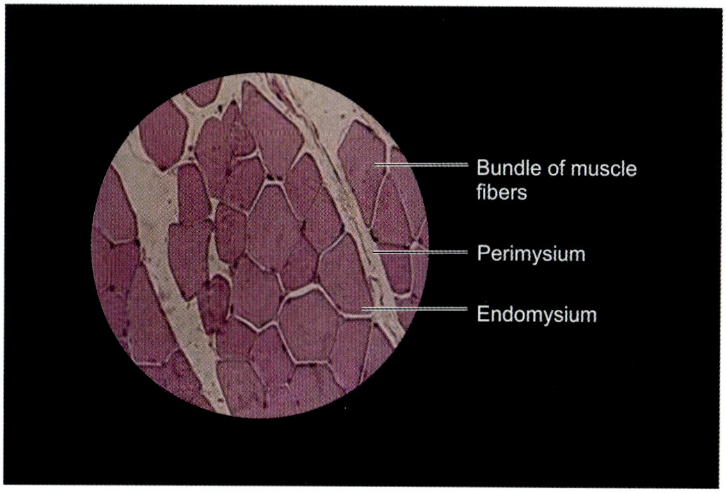

Fig. 2.29 Skeletal muscle (TS)

Blank space for sketch work by students

CARDIAC MUSCLE (FIG. 2.30)

- Cardiac muscle or myocardium is exclusively present in heart.
- They are **striated** involuntary long cylindrical cells with one or two nuclei centrally located.
- The ends of the fibers are split longitudinally to form **branches**.
- The fibers possess same arrangement of actin and myosin filaments, thus show A and I band and Z disc.
- Between the ends of adjacent cardiac muscle cells, there are specialized junctions, called **intercalated discs**.
- They provide anchorage to myofibrils and permit rapid spread of contractile stimulus from one cell to another. Hence, all fibers are triggered to contract simultaneously and functions as syncytium.
- In certain areas cardiac muscle cells modify to function as pacemakers and ramify as purkinje system.
- The red brown color in some cells is wear and tear pigment, lipofuscin.
- Cardiac muscle cells **cannot regenerate** if damaged, because they **lack satellite cells**.

Keys for identification: Cardiac muscle (LS)

a. Long cylindrical muscle fibers faintly striated and anastomosis with each other.
b. Centrally placed nucleus with perinuclear halo.
c. Intercalated disc present.

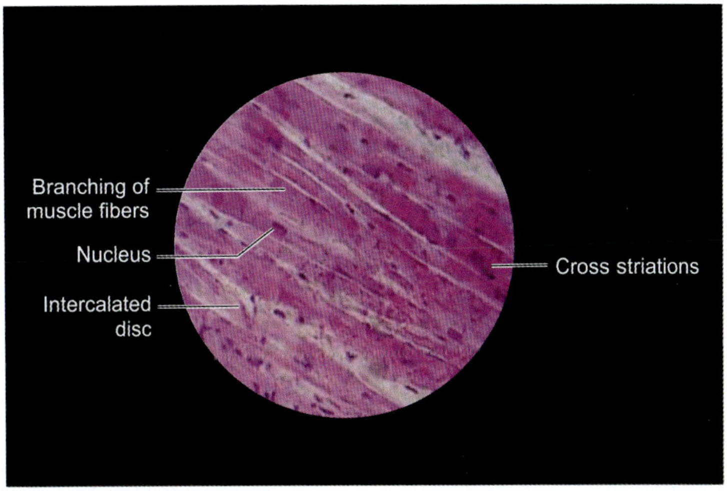

Fig. 2.30 Cardiac muscle (LS)

Blank space for sketch work by students

SMOOTH MUSCLE (FIG. 2.31)

- These are **nonstriated** and **involuntary** muscles.
- They are supplied by autonomic nervous system.
- Cells are relatively small, fusiform with single nucleus present in the center.
- The ends are tapering.
- The cells are bound together for functional requirements.

- They are seen in the wall of the hollow tubular viscera, vessels, ciliary body, iris, arrector pili muscle, etc.
- Striations are not seen.
- Contractions are of low force producing diffuse movements.
- Cells can undergo hyperplasia and hypertrophy.

Keys for identification: Smooth muscle LS and TS

a. Fibers stained deeply than surrounding connective tissue and no striations.
b. Nucleus flat oval centrally placed.
c. Long spindle shaped myocytes in bundles.

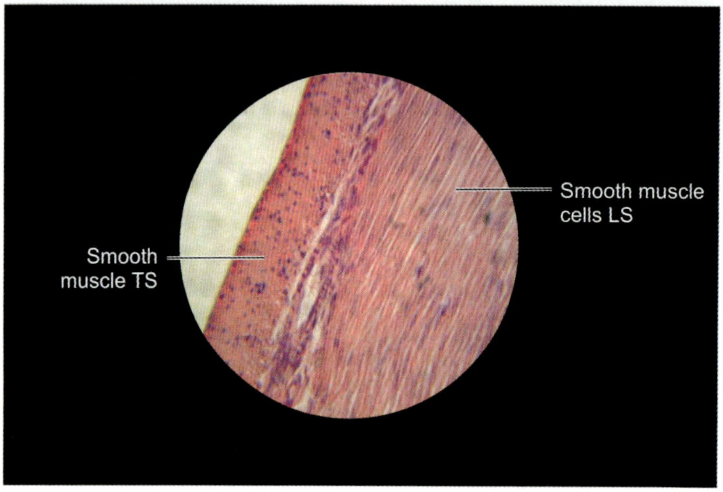

Fig. 2.31 Smooth muscle LS and TS

Blank space for sketch work by students

Comparison of Skeletal, Cardiac and Smooth Muscles

Characteristics	*Skeletal muscle*	*Cardiac muscle*	*Smooth muscle*
Location	Usually attached to bones	Present exclusively in heart	Wall of hollow viscerae, trachea, bronchi, iris and ciliary body of eye, blood vessels, arrector pili muscle of hair follicle
Fibers			
Shape	Unbranched thick, cylindrical	Branched cylindrical	Spindle shaped, small
Nucleus	Multinucleated and flat, placed peripheral beneath sarcolemma	Single in each myocyte placed centrally with perinuclear halo	Single nucleus placed centrally
Striations	Prominent transverse striations (light and dark bands)	Faint transverse striations	Striations not seen
Filament ratio	Six thin/one thick	Six thin/one thick	Twelve thin/one thick
T-tubules	At A-I band junctions form triads	At Z lines form dyads	None
Connective tissue	Organized in the form of endomysium, epimysium and perimysium	Endomysium only	Endomysium only
Junction between fibers	No junctional complex present between adjacent muscle fiber	Intercalated disc contains fascia adherens, desmosomes and gap junctions	Gap junctions are present in single unit (visceral) smooth muscle
Motor end plate	Present	Absent	Absent
Motor control	Voluntary	Involuntary	Involuntary
Nervous control	Innervated by somatic nervous system	Innervated by autonomic nervous system	Innervated by autonomic nervous system

CHAPTER

3 Systemic Histology

INTEGUMENTARY SYSTEM

It forms the largest organ and external covering of the body. It is 15–20% of the total mass and consists mainly of 3 layers.

1. Epidermis comprising of keratinized squamous epithelium which grows continuously to maintain the thickness by desquamation and is derived from ectoderm. It has the regenerating power.
2. Dermis is derived from mesoderm. It consists of dense connective tissue which provides mechanical support, strength and nourishes the fibroelastic tissue. It is divided into the papillary and reticular layers. The papillary layer is made up of the thin fine interlacing collagen fibers blood vessels, lymphatics, capillary loops and sensory nerve endings whereas the reticular layer consist of irregular collagen and elastic fibers and fibroblasts which lay these fibers, lymphocytes and macrophages and blood vessels may be found in deeper levels of the dermis. Since the skin does not have a very high metabolic demand for nutrients and oxygen, this rich vascular network serves mainly for regulation of body temperature which depends on the amount of blood flowing through superficial capillaries that allows for either conservation or dissipation of body heat.

   Arteriovenous shunts, controlled by associated sphincters, allow blood to bypass capillaries and flow directly from arteries into veins. These shunts occur in both deep and superficial dermis. In the dermis of finger tips, nose, external ear which are prone to excessive cold, AV shunts are controlled by glomus bodies which are highly convoluted portions of AV shunts surrounded by condensed collagen tissue causing thickening of vessel wall and smooth muscle cells assume an epithelioid appearance.
3. Hypodermis contains fatty tissue arranged into lobules separated by connective tissue and is equivalent to subcutaneous fascia.

FUNCTIONS OF SKIN

- Protection against mechanical, chemical, thermal, UV rays and microorganisms.
- Checks dehydration by preventing water loss.
- Maintains homeostasis.
- Helps in the regulation of body temperature. In winters hair and subcutaneous fat act as insulators and prevent heat loss. In summers it facilitates the heat loss by evaporation and keeps the surface cool.

- Synthesis of vitamin D.
- Largest sensory organ as it has receptors for touch, pain and pressure (Figs 3.1 and 3.2).

SKIN APPENDAGES

- Hair
- Sweat gland
- Sebaceous gland
- Nails
- Mammary gland.

Glomus bodies which are the highly convoluted portions in the walls of arteries, veins or AV shunts which are thickened and smooth muscle cells acquire an epithelioid appearance, concerned with temperature regulation.

Color of the skin depends on:

- Melanin.
- Oxyhemoglobin present in the dermis.
- Carotene gives yellow hue taken from the food.
- Hemosiderin golden brown in color.
- Bilirubin yellowish brown so yellow discoloration in jaundice.

CELLS OF EPIDERMIS

Four types of cells are there.

Keratinocytes

They are the predominant cells which arise in the basal layer.

Function is to produce keratin which is the major structural protein of epidermis and forms epidermal water barrier.

Melanocytes

- Present in the basal layer.
- They synthesize and release a brown pigment called melanin responsible for the color of the skin.
- Melanoblasts are derived from neural crest which give rise to melanocytes.
- Melanocytes synthesize melanin which is a brown pigment.
- Cytoplasm contains special membrane bound oval granules called premelanosome and melanosomes.
- Tyrosine is converted to DOPA which polymerizes into melanin bound to the protein.
- This melanin is transferred to basal and stratum spinosum along the cytoplasmic processes.
- Melanin secretion increases when exposed to UV rays.
- Melanin increases in the presence of UV light and this has a protective role.

- In old age melanin decreases so more chances of cancer. In albinos there is lack of tyrosinase enzyme which converts tyrosine to melanin so there is no pigment in the skin and hair.
- Melanin pigment increases in cases of hormonal imbalance in Addison's disease.

Langerhan's Cells

Langerhan's cells present in all the layers of epidermis.

- Also occur around blood vessels in papillary dermis.
- Nucleus is oval, reniform or irregular surrounded by pale cytoplasm extending as processes between keratinocytes.
- They contain rod like Berbeck granules, the ends of which distends in a vesicle resembling a tennis racket.
- They are antigen presenting cells.

Merkel Cells

Merkel cells are specialized touch receptors

- Scattered among the cells of the basal layers.
- At their bases are neuroendocrinal vesicles and have a synaptic junction with a fine nerve ending in the papillary dermis.

The layers of epidermis are best seen in thick skin. Epidermis is lined by stratified squamous keratinized epithelium and shows the following layers:

Stratum basale is the germinal layer and it shows mitotic activity (also takes place in stratum spinosum). Cells are columnar, forms a single layer which is separated from the dermis by basement membrane bounded by hemidesmosomes and provides a constant supply of keratin to replace the cells lost by normal wear and tear from 25 to 50 days.

Stratum spinosum also called **prickle cell** layer. The cells are large polyhedral and have numerous cytoplasmic processes (prickles) which show cytoplasmic basophilia and prominent nucleoli which is indicative of active protein synthesis.

Stratum granulosum cells have numerous basophilic keratohyalin granules.

Stratum lucidum is the subdivision of stratum corneum, found only in thick skin, highly refractile, nucleus and cytoplasmic organelle become disrupted and disappear as cells fill with keratin.

Stratum corneum consists of dead or dying cells. Cells are flattened, no nuclei and other organelles. Cells are filled with mature keratin.

Keys for identification: Thin skin

a. Thickness depends on the thickness of stratum corneum which is thin.
b. Absence of stratum lucidum.
c. Contains hair follicles and the epidermal ridges are less prominent.
d. Numerous arteriovenous anastomoses are there which help in thermoregulation by controlling the blood flow to dermis.
e. Thin skin is seen in the eyelids and anterior abdominal wall.

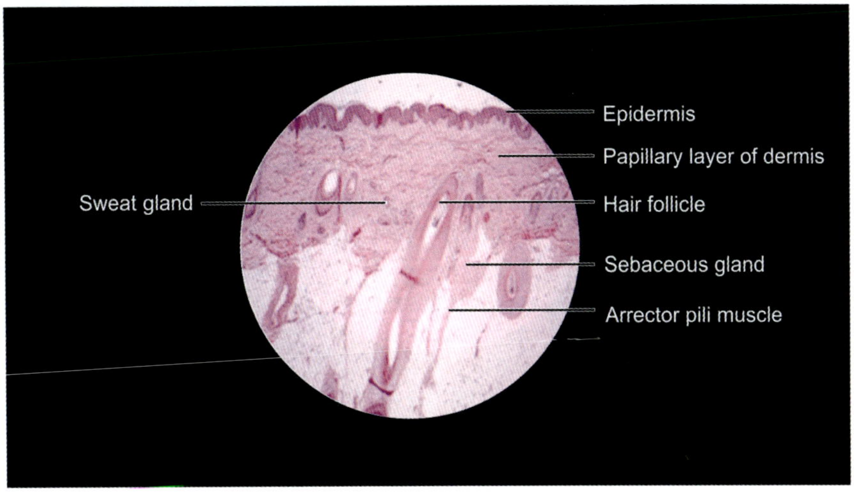

Fig. 3.1 Thin skin

Blank space for sketch work by students

- The duct is lined by stratified cuboidal epithelium (two-layered).
- Cells of duct are stained more intensely than those of the secretory portion of the gland. As fluid flows through the duct, its composition is modified by reabsorption of certain elements from the fluid. This is a means of conserving salt.
- Sweat glands are vital for thermoregulation. They also influence water and ion balance.
- The primary function for sweating is cooling of the body by evaporation. Thus, the amount of sweat is regulated as a function of body temperature. However, sweat also contains salt. Normally, sweat which comes out on the surface of the skin has a lower salt concentration than the precursor fluid produced by the secretory cells of the sweat gland. Salt is reabsorbed by the duct of the sweat gland. The effectiveness of this salt reabsorption is regulated by aldosterone the hormone responsible for maintaining electrolyte homeostasis in response to salt balance of body.

Apocrine

- Glands are present in the axillary, pubic, and perianal regions.
- Large glands that produce a viscid milky secretion.
- They do not become functional until puberty and they always secrete via a duct into the hair follicle.
- They are coiled tubular glands with a wide dilated lumen.
- Both types of sweat glands have the same basic shape, but apocrine glands have taller cells and much larger diameter.

SEBACEOUS GLAND

- Found in dermis of skin.
- Keeps skin smooth to prevent it from drying.
- Simple acinar gland whose duct usually open into hair follicle and in lips, glans penis and clitoris it directly opens on the epidermal surface with holocrine mode of secretion
- Acini consist of a layer of flat epithelial cells resting on a basement membrane.
- These are rounded cells with central nucleus and filled with fat droplets.
- Secretes sebum which is an oily secretion with antifungal and antibacterial properties.
- Secretion is controlled by testosterone in males and by androgens (ovarian and adrenal) in females.

IMMUNE SYSTEM

THE TONSILS (FIG. 3.3)

It is a special variety of lymphoid tissue which is neither primary nor secondary.

Microanatomy

It shows the presence of a **hemicapsule** on the basal side separating it from underlying muscles. The surface of the tonsils is covered by stratified squamous epithelium (nonkeratinized) which dips into the surface **forming tonsillar crypts**.

Numerous **lymphatic nodules** (B lymphocytes) are present in the lamina propria which may be primary or secondary. T lymphocytes are present in the interfollicular region.

If secondary, that is exposed to an antigen shows lighter staining germinal center with large lymphoblasts and plasma cells. At the periphery the lymphocytes are small with condensed nuclei.

The lymphocytes invade or penetrate the epithelium and come in the lumen of the crypts.

Serous and mucous acini with ducts opening on the side of crypt are seen.

Salivary corpuscles formed of desquamated epithelial cells with lymphocytes migrating through the epithelium and few bacteria.

Keys for identification: Palatine tonsil

a. Surface is covered by nonkeratinized stratified epithelium.
b. Deep to the epithelium numerous lymphoid nodules are seen.
c. Crypts are seen.

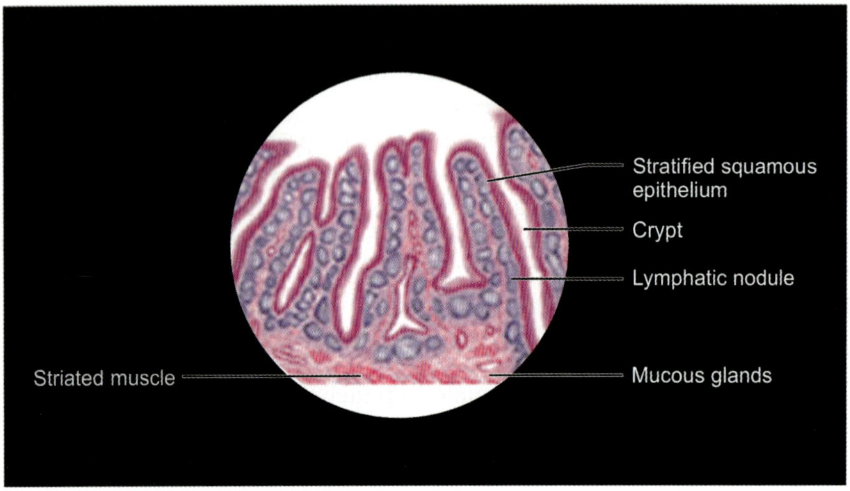

Fig. 3.3 Palatine tonsil

Blank space for sketch work by students

THYMUS (FIG. 3.4)

Its function is to produce immunologically competent T lymphocytes. From here they migrate to other tissues to populate T dependent portions of lymph node, spleen and loose connective tissue. It has no afferent lymphatics.

It is a primary lymphoreticular organ and produces a lymphocyte stimulating hormone called thymosin which increases the response to antigens and is responsible for maturation and proliferation of T lymphocytes. It involutes at puberty.

It has a thin outer fibrous covering called capsule made of elastic and collagen fibers. Thymus is of endodermal orgin, the tissue framework is formed by **epithelioreticular cells**.

From the capsule extend thin connective tissue septae (only up to corticomedullary junction) which divide it into incomplete lobules, it is only the cortex, as the medulla is a continuously branching mass surrounded by cortex. **Incomplete lobulation** is the feature of thymus. Numerous small arteries enter via septae and branch at the corticomedullary junction where the **postcapillary venules** have a special cuboidal endothelium to supply cortex and medulla.

The cortex contains an increased population of lymphocytes which are small rounded and darkly stained called **thymocytes**. Outer cortex contains large lymphocytes which divide by mitosis into small lymphocyte which are pushed deeper into the medulla. Only few lymphocytes leave the thymus via post capillary venules in the medulla as immunocompetent T lymphocytes and majority die in the thymus because they act against self antigen of the body. The process of maturation includes proliferation rearrangement of T-cell receptor (TCR) genes to produce a large variety of specific antigens and acquiring surface markers (phenotypes) of T-cells, i.e. mature helper and cytotoxic T-cells. At this stage, T-cells which react against self antigens (normal body components) are removed by apoptosis and establish self tolerance. The dead cells are taken up by pale stained macrophages at the corticomedullary junction giving a starry sky appearance.

Epithelioreticular cells are flattened, pale staining, supporting cells called **epitheliocytes**. It gives out cellular processes which are branched and are bounded together by desmosomes and lie in close contact with adjoining cells forming a membrane or a barrier called hemothymic barrier which is made up of endothelial lining of capillaries, little perivascular space and epithelial lining formed by epithelioreticular cells. The barrier prevents exposure of the immature lymphocytes to blood borne antigens. These epitheliocytes also form a framework for the lymphocytes. Cortical epithelial cells called nurse cell surround many lymphocytes promoting T-cell differentiation and proliferation. They also secrete at least four peptide hormones named as thymulin, thymopoietin, alpha and beta thymosin that regulate and promote T-cell maturation and proliferation.

Medulla is similar to the germinal center of lymphatic organ which is lightly stained. It contains several **Hassall's corpuscles** which are oval or spherical whorl like aggregation of flattened **Type VI epithelioreticular cells** arranged concentrically and contain pink eosinophilic degenerating material in the center. The center of the corpuscle shows keratinization. The young thymus is more cellular with less adipose tissue in between the lobules.

There are no afferent lymphatic vessels so it cannot react to circulating antigens, it has only efferent lymphatics.

Keys for identification: Thymus

a. Capsule sends trabeculae in the cortex only forming leaf like lobule.
b. Cortex is composed of small darkly stained lymphocytes, epitheliocytes and macrophages.
c. In the medulla Hassall's corpuscles are seen.

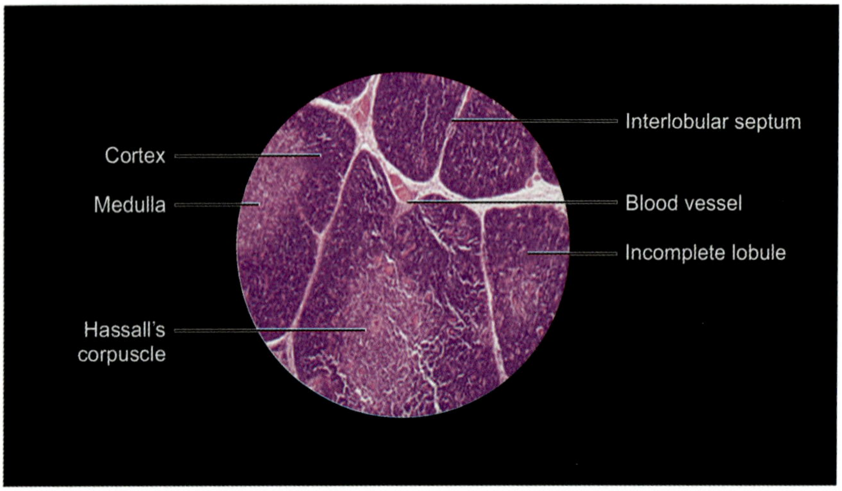

Fig. 3.4 Thymus

Blank space for sketch work by students

LYMPH NODE (FIG. 3.5)

The Lymph Node is a collection of lymphatic tissue organized to form an organ.

It consists of a capsule formed by dense collagen and elastic fibers.

The **capsule** sends processes known as **trabeculae** into the substance of the node which form incomplete septa.

Between the capsule and the substance of the node is present a space called **subcapsular sinus** into which the afferent lymphatics open. The substance of the node has a coarse framework formed by the reticular fibers which are more closely set in the cortex than in the medulla.

On the reticular mesh is present the cellular stroma which exists as rounded or pear shaped zones in the cortex called **cortical nodules**. The cortical nodules may be primary or secondary. A primary nodule has no germinal center which exists only in secondary nodule which is a reaction center in response to an antigen.

The germinal center is lightly stained area containing large lymphocytes and plasma cells. It is considered as zone 3, dark rims of the follicle as zone 2. The term zone 1 is applied to the region immediately around the follicle containing loosely packed lymphocytes, plasma cells and macrophages. Zone 1 becomes continuous with the medullary cords.

In between the cortex (has B lymphocytes) and the medulla is the **paracortex** which contains (T lymphocytes). Paracortex lies between the cortical nodules and the medulla. It is densely cellular, homogenous but few nodules may be seen in the deeper paracortex. The venules in the paracortex comprise important entry points for the lymphocytes from the blood into the lymph node (90%). A few (10%) lymphocytes also enter from lymph vessels.

The **medulla** consists of:

- Medullary cords which are the extensions of the lymphatic tissue arising from the cortex and paracortex containing both B lymphocytes, T lymphocytes, plasma cells and macrophages.
- Medullary sinuses which are continuous with cortical sinuses join together at the hilus to deliver lymph to efferent lymphatic vessel.

Flow of lymph afferent vessels cross the capsule and pour lymph into the subcapsular sinus, cortical sinuses, medullary sinuses and efferent vessels. Due to valves in both afferent and efferent vessels there is unidirectional flow of blood. During this passage lymph infiltrates the cortex and medullary cords where it is filtered and modified by immune cells.

Keys for identification: Lymph node

a. Presence of capsule and subcapsular sinus.
b. In the cortex are present lymphatic nodules.
c. Medulla shows medullary cords and sinuses.

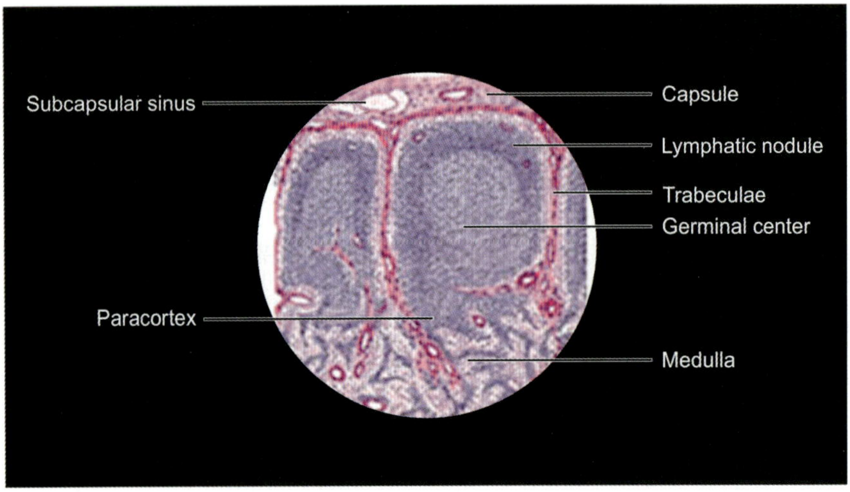

Fig. 3.5 Lymph node

Blank space for sketch work by students

SPLEEN (FIG. 3.6)

Spleen is a lymphoid organ associated with the blood vascular system. Its function is to screen the blood and thus helps in immunological response.

B lymphocytes in the spleen are exposed to antigens present in circulating blood.

The blood (especially the RBCs) in the spleen can be returned to the circulation rapidly in an emergency, so acts as a reservoir of blood.

The spleen is covered by a capsule consisting of dense fibroelastic connective tissue, some smooth muscle, and an outer covering of mesothelium. Trabecular extensions of the capsule (which contain blood vessels) partially subdivide the spleen. The parenchymal tissue is supported on a framework of reticular connective tissue and **is not differentiated into cortex and medulla.**

Two types of parenchymal tissue can be identified in the spleen.

White Pulp

White pulp consists of typical dense lymphoid tissue organized around arterial vessels as periarterial lymphoid sheaths (PALS). The central "artery" in a PALS is really an arteriole. Most of the inner cells of PALS are recirculating T-cells, but nodules containing B lymphocytes also occur. White pulp is composed of splenic nodule which is traversed by the central arteriole but is eccentric in position because they avoid the germinal center where the B lymphocytes are produced.

Red Pulp

Red pulp is located between white pulp and trabeculae. It contains small arteries called penicilli, capillaries, venous sinuses, and diffuse lymphoid tissue in the form of cords (cords of Billroth). Other cells seen are reticular cells, lymphocytes, macrophages, monocytes, plasma cells and granular leukocytes and erythrocytes. The central artery gives a number of branches called penicillar arteries at right angles and terminate as sheathed capillaries which form first part of filtering mechanism of spleen. These are unique vessels which have no endothelial lining and surrounded by a thickening of macrophages, forming the ellipsoid arteriole whose distal part is dilated to form the ampulla which open in the reticular framework of splenic cords (open circulation) or directly into the venous sinusoids from where the blood is drained into the venules and then into the veins which come out of the hilum (closed circulation). Passage of blood through the spleen is complex.

Trabecular arteries → arterioles of white pulp smaller arterioles → capillaries of red pulp → venous sinuses in red pulp → trabecular veins.

Venous sinusoids are lined by large cells which bulge into the lumen called **stave cells**. These cells are wrapped by reticular fibers set in transverse direction. These sinusoids are surrounded by an incomplete basal lamina. **Stave cells** have a unique property that allows only healthy red blood cells to enter but the aged red blood cells (senesence antigen) undergoes changes in the membrane which gets swollen and is less flexible so they do not enter in the sinusoids.

Perilymphoid zone of red pulp just outside white pulp differs from red pulp by absence of sinuses, very few reticulin fibers and a large number of RBCs and WBCs (10%) of blood in spleen which passes very slowly in the sinuses of red pulp. This sluggish blood flow increases the interaction of blood cells antigens and antibodies.

Macrophages in the spleen remove old, abnormal, and damaged blood cells from the blood by phagocytosis.

Keys for identification: Spleen

a. Capsule sends trabeculae in the parenchyma (not differentiated into cortex and medulla).
b. White pulp shows lymphoid follicles with eccentric arteriole (Malpighian corpuscle).
c. Highly vascular red pulp surrounds the white pulp.

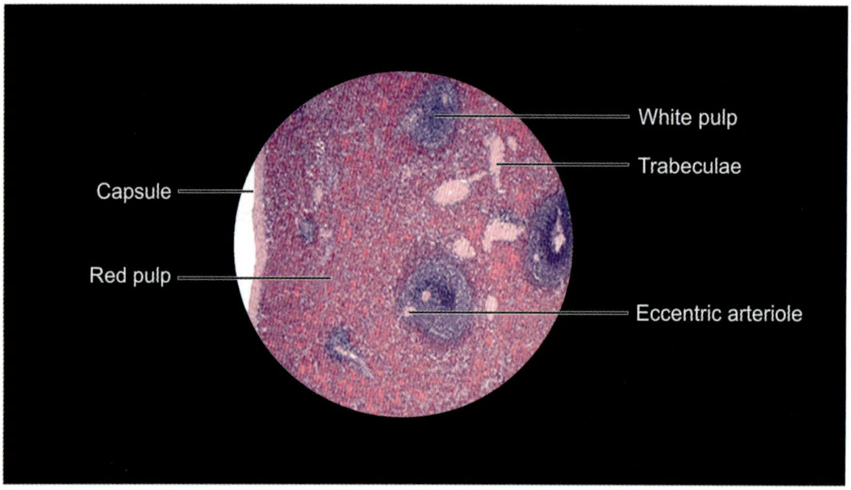

Fig. 3.6 Spleen

Blank space for sketch work by students

Features of Important Tissues/Organs

Tissue/Organ	*Capsule*	*Cortex-Medulla*	*Germinal Centers*	*Lobulation*
Tonsils	Yes on one side, Covered on other side by stratified squamous epithelium (SSE)	No	Yes	Infoldings of SSE and underlying CT form tonsillar crypts
Lymph node	Yes	Yes	Yes	No. Framework contains trabeculae which are elongated dense CT spicules extending from capsule
Thymus	Yes	Yes	No (Hassall's corpuscle represents germinal center)	Yes. Cortex is partially lobulated by septae (dense CT walls), where as medulla is continuous
Spleen	Yes may have smooth muscle fibers no subcapsular sinus	No Nodules spread throughout organ	Yes	No. Framework contains trabeculae, elongated dense CT spicules extending from capsule

Muscular arteries are the distributing vessels and control the amount of blood flowing through them (Fig. 3.8).

- All the named arteries in the body, except for the large elastic arteries, are muscular arteries. The thickness of the wall is usually more than the diameter of lumen.

  T. intima consists of endothelium, a flattened subendothelial layer of collagenous fibers and internal elastic lamina is very prominent and wavy.
- The media is the major identifying features. It consists of a thick smooth muscle layer with as many as 40 layers of smooth muscle encircling the lumen.
- Larger muscular arteries may have a prominent external elastic lamina at the border of the media with the adventitia.
- Adventitia is well developed and usually thinner than media.
- Spasmodic contraction of the media smooth muscle helps prevent bleeding.
- Lumen is circular.
- Prominent internal elastic lamina is thrown into wavy folds.
- Tunica media is thick and muscular (circularly arranged smooth muscles)
- Well developed external elastic lamina.

Keys for identification: Arteries

a. Lumen is small, patent, round and thick walled.
b. Well defined endothelial lining with distinct internal and external lamina.
c. T. media forms 2/3rd of the thickness of the wall.
d. T. adventitia is thin forms 1/3rd of thickness of wall.
e. Contain oxygenated blood except pulmonary and umbilical arteries.
f. No blood is seen in the lumen.
g. Vasa vasorum supply nutrition up to outer 2/3rd of T. media.
h. Valves are absent.

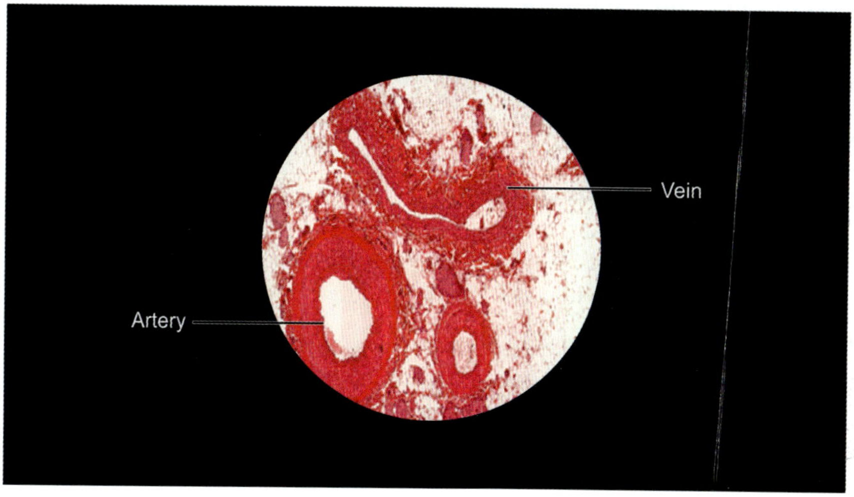

Fig. 3.10 Comparison between artery and vein

Blank space for sketch work by students

RESPIRATORY SYSTEM

The respiratory system has two parts:

1. The **conducting** part includes nasal cavity, nasopharynx, bronchus, bronchioles up to terminal bronchioles.
2. The **respiratory** part includes respiratory bronchioles, alveolar duct, alveolar sac and the alveoli.

FUNCTIONS OF THE RESPIRATORY SYSTEM

- Exchange of gases
- Regulation of blood pH
- It has sensory function as it has small receptors
- Filters and conditions the inspired air
- Larynx helps in the voice production.

Epiglottis (Fig. 3.11)

It is a thin leaf like plate of elastic cartilage.

Microanatomy

Structurally consists of:

- Central core of elastic cartilage.
- Both the surfaces of cartilage are covered by mucous membrane which consists of :
  - Stratified squamous nonkeratinized epithelium on oral side.
  - Pseudostratified columnar ciliated on laryngeal side.
- Lamina propria or the subepithelial connective tissue contains plenty of elastic fibers, both serous and mucous glands and few taste buds on the oral surface.

Keys for identification: Epiglottis

a. Elastic cartilage in the middle.
b. Stratified squamous epithelium on one surface.
c. Pseudostratified ciliated columnar epithelium on the other surface.

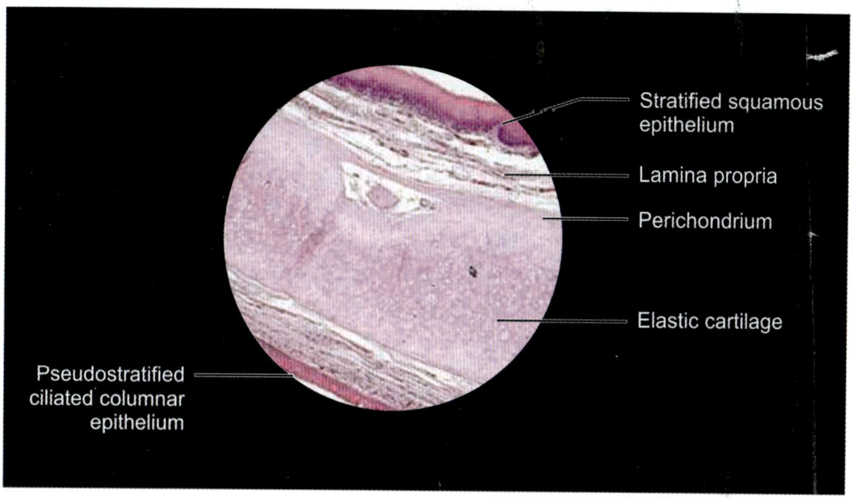

Fig. 3.11 Epiglottis

Blank space for sketch work by students

TRACHEA (FIG. 3.12)

It is a flexible tube which permits expansion in diameter and length during inspiration and passive recoil during expiration.

Microanatomy

It consists of innermost layer of mucous membrane which is having an epithelium and lamina propria. Epithelium is lined by **pseudostratified ciliated columnar** epithelium having three types of cells.

1. **Tall columnar ciliated** cells, each having about 250 cilia with a basal body which sweeps the mucus from further places to the pharynx.
2. **Goblet cells** secrete mucus which traps the bacteria and other particulate matter and removes it from the inspired air. The term goblet refers to shape of the cell as the apical part is filled with mucus and displaces the nucleus towards the base.
3. Small columnar cells which rest on the basement membrane and do not reach up to the lumen, and act as a **stem or the reserve** cells which replace the damaged mucosa.

Lamina propria has numerous seromucous glands.

There is no muscularis mucosae, if present then it is in the form of elastic fibers between mucosa and submucosa.

- Inner to this is the **cartilage** which is **hyaline** in nature, made up of 16–20 rings (replaced by bone in old age) called tracheal ring which are in the form of incomplete C shaped and deficient posteriorly. The gap between the posterior ends of the rings is bridged by the smooth muscle fibers called **trachealis** muscle which relaxes during swallowing to facilitate the passage of large pieces of food by allowing esophagus to bulge into the lumen of trachea with the elastic layer preventing excessive distension of lumen. But during the cough reflex muscle contracts to narrow the tracheal lumen to increase the velocity of expelled air thus loosening of materials in the air passage.
- **Thick basement membrane** characteristic of tracheal epithelium is due to increased collagen fiber bundles which lie between basal lamina and coarse reticular lamina. In smokers and in chronic cough it is very thick in response to the mucosal irritation.
- Lamina propria is rich in diffuse lymphoid tissue which infiltrates the mucosa and the submucosa functionally equivalent to BALT (bronchus associated lymphatic tissue).

Keys for identification: Trachea

a. Epithelium lined by pseudostratified columnar ciliated epithelium.
b. Serous and mucous acini present.
c. C shaped hyaline cartilage seen.

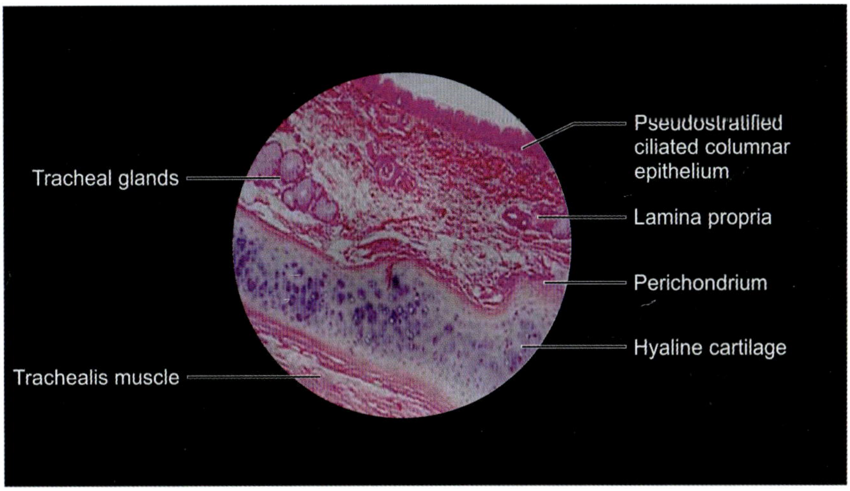

Fig. 3.12 Trachea

Blank space for sketch work by students

Extrapulmonary bronchus

It is histologically same as trachea.

LUNGS (FIG. 3.13)

Intrapulmonary Bronchus

Cartilaginous rings are replaced by cartilage plates of irregular shape and disappear where the airway reaches a diameter of 1 mm in the bronchioles.
There are five layers:

1. Mucosa consist of pseudostratified tall columnar ciliated epithelium with goblet cells but it is less tall and lamina propria is more dense with large quantity of elastic fibers in superficial part with seromucinous glands.
2. Muscularis mucosa is a continuous layer of smooth muscles.
3. Submucosa consists of glands and adipose tissue present in large bronchi.
4. A layer of hyaline cartilage present as plates.
5. Adventitia is a layer of dense connective tissue.

Lobular Bronchiole

When the diameter of a bronchus becomes 1 mm or less it is called **bronchiole**, characterized by:

- No cartilage and no glands in the mucosa.
- Gradual diminution in the height of the epithelium which becomes columnar first and then finally cuboidal.
- Goblet cells may be seen in lobular bronchiole but in terminal and respiratory bronchiole goblet cells are replaced by **clara** cells.

Terminal Bronchioles

They are the smallest diameter passages of the conducting system characterized by no cartilage, no glands, no goblet cells and the lining epithelium is ciliated simple columnar or cuboidal where the clara cells are interspersed between ciliated cells.

Respiratory Bronchiole

Mucosa is structurally similar to terminal bronchiole, i.e. lined by ciliated low columnar to cuboidal epithelium and few nonciliated clara cells except their walls contain small number of single alveoli.

Functions of Clara Cells

- Produce components of surfactant.
- Act as reserve cell, i.e. divide, differentiate and replace the damaged cell types.
- Contain enzymes that detoxify noxious or harmful substances.

Alveolar Duct

They are elongated passages having numerous alveoli opening along their length, i.e. their walls are made up of alveoli. A ring of smooth muscle, collagen and elastic fibers is formed around the opening of alveolar duct, alveolar sac and alveoli to regulate air movements. Alveolar septum is formed between adjacent alveoli and can be compared to a sandwich, in which bread is formed by two layers of basement membrane of adjacent alveoli and filling by capillaries, elastin and collagen fibers. This alveolar septum also contains numerous pores which equalize the pressure between alveoli and provide a collateral passage.

Alveoli

They are small pockets that are open on one side. The alveolar wall consists of three components:
1. The alveolar epithelium.
2. Supporting tissue between epithelium and surrounding blood vessel of the alveolar wall, consists of fine reticular, collagen and elastic fibers and occasional fibroblasts.
3. Blood vessels are mainly capillaries. In most of the alveolar wall basement membrane of capillaries is directly applied to the basement membrane of alveolar cells with no supporting tissue so there is minimal thickness interface between air and blood.

Alveolar Epithelium Consists of the following Cell Types

- **Type I pneumocytes** are large squamous cells for gaseous exchange. About 95% of alveolar surface is lined by these cells.
- **Type II pneumocytes** are cuboidal cells which have large rounded nuclei with prominent nucleolus and vacuolated cytoplasm which secretes surfactant which prevents the collapse of alveoli in expansion. They also retain the capacity for cell division and can differentiate into Type I in response to damage of alveolar lining. Surfactant is also secreted by **Clara cells** of respiratory bronchioles which synthesize the other components of surfactant. These cells are characterized by membrane bound lamellar bodies which store pulmonary surfactant.
- **Type III** alveolar cells or **Brush cells** are columnar cells without cilia but have abundant apical microvilli. They have sensory function of smell and monitor the quality of air and do not contain any secretory granules.
- Granular cells (**Kulchitsky cells**) which contain abundant secretory granules below the nuclei and contain a variety of hormones. They represent the enteroendocrine cells of gut and their presence is explained by being derived from the same endodermal layer same as basal cells.
- Some carbon particles reach the alveoli and are engulfed by alveolar macrophages which are large phagocytic cells derived from the blood monocytes found in the alveolar wall or in the alveolar space.
- **Heart failure** cells are large monocytes derived from mononuclear system which phagocytose blood cells and cellular debris entering the alveoli as a result of heart failure.

Keys for identification: Lung

a. Numerous thin walled empty spaces (Honeycomb appearance of alveoli).
b. Lining endothelium (simple squamous epithelium).
c. Intrapulmonary bronchi, bronchioles and respiratory bronchioles are seen.

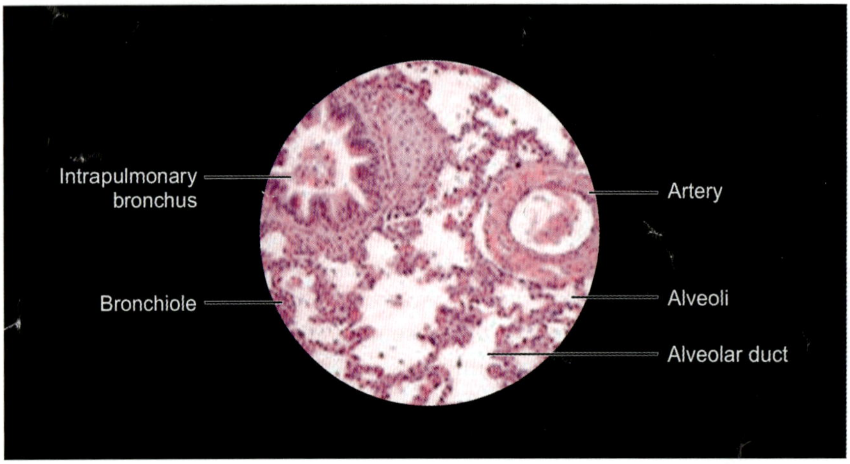

Fig. 3.13 Lung

Blank space for sketch work by students

Differences between Bronchus and Bronchiole

Bronchus	*Bronchiole*
Diameter is more compared to bronchiole	Diameter is less compared to bronchi
Lined by pseudostratified ciliated epithelium with goblet cells	Large size bronchiole is lined by simple columnar cells with few cilia and goblet cells. Small size bronchiole is lined with simple columnar or simple cuboidal cells with no cilia or goblet cells
Smooth muscle layer between mucosa and cartilage layer not well-defined	Smooth muscle and elastic fibers form a well-defined layer beneath mucosa
Cartilage is present as irregular plates	Cartilage is absent
Mucous and serous acini are present between muscle and cartilage layer in submucosa	No glands seen in submucosa

Differences between Extrapulmonary and Intrapulmonary Bronchus

	Extrapulmonary bronchus	*Intrapulmonary bronchus*
Mucous Membrane	Thrown into folds posteriorly	Thrown into folds throughout the lumen because of a complete layer of muscle between the cartilage and the mucous membrane
Glands	Lie between mucous membrane and cartilage	Lie between cartilage and muscle
Muscle	Present posteriorly	Forms a complete layer beneath the mucous membrane
Cartilage	C-shaped	Irregular and in many pieces

SALIVARY GLANDS

A gland is a structure that produces a secretion necessary for normal body functioning. They are of two types—exocrine and endocrine.

MAJOR PAIRED SALIVARY GLANDS

- Parotid gland
- Submandibular gland
- Sublingual gland.

MINOR GLANDS

- Labial
- Von Ebner's gland.

They produce saliva which is a mixed secretion, derived from large and small salivary glands. Salivation is regulated by parasympathetic nervous system.

FUNCTIONS OF SALIVA

- Saliva (water) moistens the oral mucosa as well as dry food before swallowing
- Mucus (lubricates food for easy swallowing).
- Its high bicarbonate content buffers the oral cavity.
- It provides a medium for food materials to stimulate taste buds.
- It begins the digestion of carbohydrates via the digestive enzyme amylase.
- It controls the bacterial flora by secreting lysozyme.
- In the absence of saliva, infections and caries would develop in the oral tissues.
- The salivary glands also secrete IgA and potassium, and reabsorb sodium.

All of these glands are *tubuloacinar glands,* i.e. they have secretory acini but the first part of the duct system arising from the acini also forms the secretory units. The salivary glands are divided by connective tissue septa into lobes, which are further subdivided into lobules.

Functionally the secretory acini can be divided into two groups (Fig. 3.14):

1. **Serous acini** secrete a liquid product, are smaller, contain a round or slightly ovoid nucleus which is placed basally in the cell. The lumen is very small. The bluish color of the basal cytoplasm shows the presence of rough endoplasmic reticulum, the apical cytoplasm may appear pinkish/red or, contain reddish granules. The granules represent the vesicles which contain the secretory product of the cell. The digestive enzyme α-amylase is also secreted by the acinar cells. Serous secretions are watery. They may be present on the mucous acini as serous demilunes.
2. **Mucous acini** secrete a very viscous product. The cells forming the mucous acini usually contain flattened nuclei which appear to be "pressed" against the basal surface of the cell, are larger and lighter than serous cell. Secretory vesicles fill much of the apical cytoplasm. The secretory product has either been dissolved during the staining process or remains unstained. Small amount of cytoplasm which remains between the vesicles give the apical part of the cell a distinct foamy appearance. Lumen is visible. They are complete acini.

In compound or mixed acini, the serous cells form small half-moon or crescent-shaped structures, which attach to mucous acini and empty their secretory product into interstices between the mucous producing cells. Looking at their appearance they are called serous demilunes.

Both serous and mucous acini and parts of the secretory duct system are surrounded by myoepithelial cells which by their contractions participate in the secretory process.

The glands present close to the mouth have mucous acini, e.g. sublingual glands further away from the oral cavity have serous secretions, e.g. parotid gland. The submandibular glands contain both serous and mucous acini but it is predominantly serous. The sublingual is predominantly mucous with serous demilunes.

Keys for identification: Serous acini

a. Cells are pyramidal in shape.
b. Apical part contains secretory granules and nucleus is displaced basally.
c. Lumen is small.

Keys for identification: Mucous acini

a. Larger size of acini.
b. Lightly stained.
c. Nucleus is flattened and present towards the base.

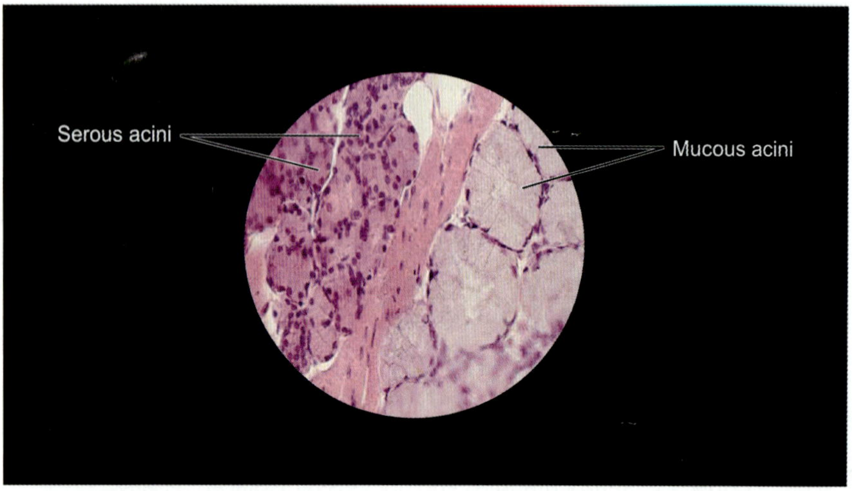

Fig. 3.14 Serous and mucous acini

Blank space for sketch work by students

DUCT SYSTEM

There are two types of ducts:

1. *Intralobular ducts* seen in the lobule. They include intercalated and striated ducts. The secretory acini merge and empty into intercalated ducts which merge into the striated ducts.
   Intercalated ducts
   - Are the smallest intralobular ducts
   - Connect individual acini to the striated ducts
   - Lined by a simple, low cuboidal epithelium which add bicarbonate ions to the saliva (buffering function) and absorb chloride from the saliva
   - Intercalated ducts are difficult to identify in mucous glands as they are very short.

Striated ducts
- Lined by columnar epithelial cells.
- The nucleus is located almost between the apical and basal cell surfaces.
- The striations are found in the basal part of the cytoplasm where numerous mitochondria are found between infoldings of the basal cell membrane.
- This specialization provides the cell with the necessary energy and surface area to perform its task in the modification of the saliva—the secretion of potassium and the reabsorption of sodium from the primary secretion.
- Cells of the striated ducts also take up a secretory form of antibodies and release them into the saliva.
- Striated ducts are absent in purely mucous glands.
- Serous cells secrete a fluid isotonic with plasma. In striated ducts ions are reabsorbed and secreted to produce hypotonic saliva containing less sodium and chloride and more potassium and bicarbonate than plasma.

2. *Interlobular ducts* are large ducts found within the dense connective tissue septa that are located between the lobules and lobes. All interlobular ducts are excretory ducts. They ultimately connect with the oral cavity. Their epithelium is variable, it can be simple cuboidal, stratified cuboidal, simple columnar, stratified columnar or pseudostratified and finally becomes stratified squamous near their opening into the oral cavity. Excretory ducts do not change the secretory product.

PAROTID GLAND (FIG. 3.15)

Microanatomy

- It is a serous gland showing serous cells.
- Well-differentiated intercalated and striated ducts are a prominent feature of the parotid gland, rare in the submandibular gland, and absent in the sublingual gland.
- Fairly large amounts of adipose tissue which is found between the secretroy tissue of the lobules aid in the identification of the parotid gland.
- As they approach the excretory ducts, their diameter may exceed that of the acini. The ducts also secrete lysozyme and IgA.

Keys for identification: Parotid gland (serous)

a. Small round basophilic serous acini are seen.
b. No serous demilunes seen.
c. Intercalated and striated ducts seen.
d. Large amount of adipose tissue is present.

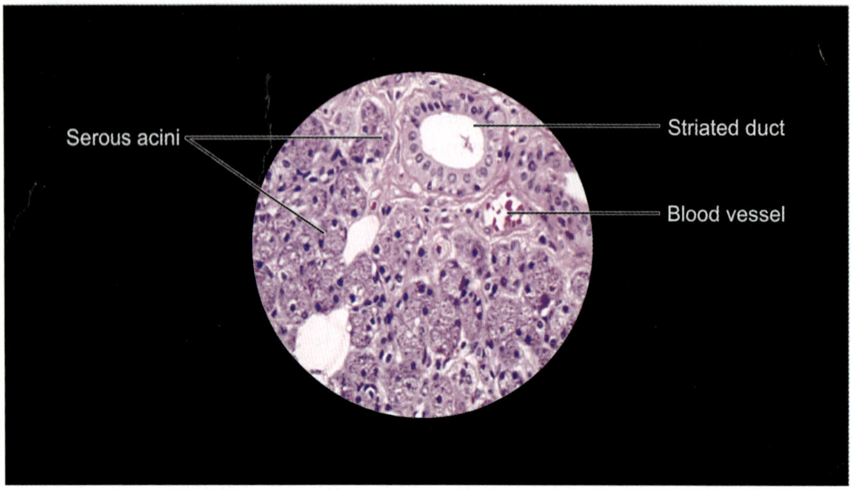

Fig. 3.15 Parotid gland (serous)

Blank space for sketch work by students

SUBMANDIBULAR GLAND (FIG. 3.16)

Microanatomy

Each acinus is round alveolar, or acinar in shape. Serous cells have a pyramidal shape and there is a spherical nucleus near the base of the cell.

They have a very basophilic cytoplasm because of many ribosomes and basophilic zymogen granules that store the serous secretory product of the cells. Mucous acini are more tubular in shape and have larger lumen than serous acini. Loose connective tissue surrounds each acinus and supports them.

Keys for identification: Submandibular gland (Mixed)

a. Both serous and mucous acini seen.
b. Acini are lined by truncated columnar cells.
c. Some serous demilunes seen.

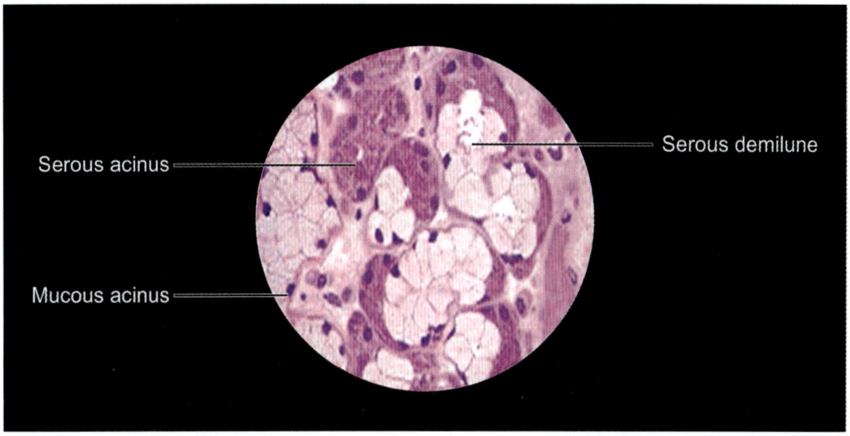

Fig. 3.16 Submandibular gland (Mixed)

Blank space for sketch work by students

SUBLINGUAL GLAND (FIG. 3.17)

Microanatomy

It contains both serous and mucous acini but mucous acini predominate.

Mucous acini have a larger lumen than serous acini. They acini are capped by serous demilune but purely serous acini are rarely present. Formation of these demilunes is actually a fixation artefact (mucous cells swell with fixation techniques and squeeze out the serous cell).

The intercalated and striated ducts are composed of flattened or low columnar epithelium but they are very short so difficult to find. Intercalated duct join with other one or more intercalated ducts to form intralobular duct which has a larger lumen and is lined by columnar cells.

Keys for identification: Sublingual gland (Mucous)

a. Large light stained mucous acini seen and pure serous acini are rare to find.
b. Typical serous demilune is seen.
c. Mainly intralobular ducts are present with very few intercalated or striated ducts.

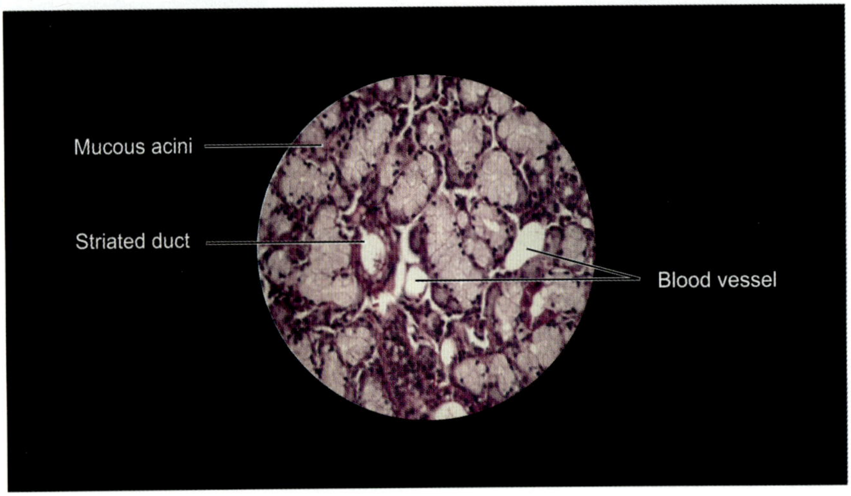

Fig. 3.17 Sublingual gland (Mucous)

Blank space for sketch work by students

THE DIGESTIVE SYSTEM

Digestive system converts the food that we eat into a form that can be processed and used as energy for all the activities carried out by the body.

Digestive system consists of two parts.

1. *Gastrointestinal tract* consists of a tube from mouth to anus.
2. *Accessory organs of digestion* include teeth, tongue, salivary glands, liver, gallbladder and pancreas.

FUNCTIONS OF DIGESTIVE SYSTEM

- *Ingestion:* Taking in of food and liquids.
- *Secretion:* Water, enzymes, acid or buffers are secreted into the gastrointestinal tract.
- *Mixing and propulsion:* Food is churned and moved along the GIT by peristalsis.
- *Digestion:* Food is mechanically and chemically broken into smaller particles.
- *Absorption:* Passage of digested substances into the gut wall and then into blood and lymph.
- *Defecation:* Elimination of undigested or unabsorbed waste in the faeces.

The process of digestion begins in the mouth. Food is taken in and chewed until it reaches a consistency in which it can be swallowed. The structures which help in digestion are as follows:

Tongue

It is a muscular structure that is covered by taste buds. It helps in chewing of food and moving it to a position from where it can be swallowed easily.

Salivary Glands

They secrete the enzyme salivary amylase which begins the process of chemical digestion by breaking down carbohydrates. Saliva also moistens food which helps it to be swallowed more easily.

Teeth

They break down food into smaller particles so that ingestion is easier.

Pharynx allows the passage of both food and air.

Esophagus

It leads to the stomach where mechanical breakdown of food occurs by the action of muscles within the digestive tract and chemical breakdown of food by enzymes is done.

Stomach

The food remains in the stomach for 3–4 hours. During this time it is further broken down by the muscular churning action of the stomach. Powerful gastric juices are also secreted by the cells of the stomach, contributing in chemical digestion and forming chyme. 10% absorption takes place in the stomach. Epithelial cells in the stomach are impermeable to most substances but absorb water, ions, short chain fatty acids, drugs (aspirin) and alcohol.

Small Intestine

Digested material is moved through the small intestine by muscular contractions called peristalsis. The process of digestion is completed in the small intestine. Absorption of substances takes place as they pass through the walls of the digestive tract into the bloodstream. 90% absorption of all nutrients takes place in the small intestine through its walls. So digestion and absorption takes place in the small intestines.

Large Intestine

The waste material then moves into the large intestine where water is reabsorbed changing it into a more solid form, ready to be excreted through the rectum. Colon secretes mucus, but no enzymes. Contraction of *Taenia coli* gathers colon into pouches called **haustrae**.

Movement of chyme in the large intestine occurs by haustral churning in which haustrae fill with chyme and then muscles contract to push chyme into next haustrum by peristalsis.

ORAL CAVITY

The oral cavity is divided in a vestibule, the area "outside" the teeth, and an oral cavity proper. The entire oral cavity is lined by a stratified squamous epithelium. The epithelial lining is divided into two broad types:

1. Masticatory epithelium is keratinized covers the surfaces involved in the processing of food (tongue, gingivae and hard plate).
2. Lining epithelium i.e. nonkeratinized stratified squamous epithelium, covers the remaining surfaces of the oral cavity protecting oral cavity from pathogens.

Tongue (Fig. 3.18)

It forms the floor of oral cavity. It places food on the teeth for chewing and helps with swallowing and speech. The dorsal surface of the tongue is divided by the sulcus terminalis into an oral part, the anterior two-thirds, and a pharyngeal part, the posterior one-third.

Microanatomy

The mucosa of the tongue consists of stratified squamous epithelium. The dorsal surface of the tongue is characterized by a large number of small projections, the lingual papillae that contain taste buds. The lingual papillae consist of a connective tissue core covered with a stratified squamous epithelium. On the basis of their appearance four types of papillae can be distinguished—filiform, fungiform, circumvallate and foliate papillae.

Filiform papillae are the smallest and most numerous papillae. By providing the tongue with a rough surface (keratinized) they aid in the manipulation and processing of foods. They do not possess taste buds.

Fungiform papillae occur singly and are fairly evenly spaced between the filiform papillae. Their connective tissue core is richly vascularized giving a red appearance. The epithelium is slightly thinner (nonkeratinized).

Circumvallate papillae are the largest 8–12 in number. They are set into the tongue's surface and surrounded with a trench formed by the infolding of the epithelium. Taste buds are particularly numerous on the lateral surfaces of these papillae. The excretory ducts of serous glands open into the trenches surrounding the papillae ("rinsing glands" or glands of von Ebner). This moat like arrangement provides a continuous flow of fluid over the taste buds to wash the food particles so that taste buds can receive and process new taste stimulus.

Foliate papillae are not well developed in humans and may be absent in aged individuals. If present, they form lamellae along the posterior and lateral border of the tongue.

In the center of tongue are present bundles of skeletal muscles running in different directions permitting great mobility for speech, chewing and swallowing.

In the lower part are seen mucous, serous and mixed acini with serous demilunes. The interlobular ducts pass into larger excretory ducts which open on the ventral surface in the mouth cavity.

TASTE BUDS (FIG. 3.19)

They lie at the bottom of a furrow. They are embedded in the stratified squamous epithelium of the circumvallate papilla. They are oval in shape, composed of three types of cells.

1. Taste or the **gustatory cell** which shows light cytoplasm with oval and lighter nucleus.
2. Supporting or the **sustentacular cells** with darker cytoplasm and slender dark nucleus.
3. **Basal cells** present at the periphery near the basement membrane.

Both gustatory and sustentacular cells have long microvilli that protrude through the taste pore.

Taste buds are washed by the secretions of von Ebner's gland.

Lamina propria is thin and papillated forming secondary papillae in fungiform and circumvallate papillae.

Seromucous glands are seen.

Muscularis externa consists of skeletal muscle fibers cut in different planes.

ESOPHAGUS (FIG. 3.20)

It is a 10" long muscular tube posterior to trachea through which food passes to the stomach.

Microanatomy

The mucosa: The lumen is lined by a thick protective stratified squamous epithelium (non-keratinized) with the stem cells scattered throughout the basal layer. It is deeply folded longitudinally (an arrangement which permits marked distension during the passage of food).

Lamina propria: The connective tissue papilla indents the epithelium and contains small blood vessels and diffuse lymphatic tissue. The mucosal glands are located luminal to the muscularis mucosae. In the part of the esophagus closest to the stomach there may be mucosal mucous-producing glands, which protect the esophageal mucosa from acidic reflux from the stomach.

Muscularis mucosae is a layer of smooth muscle fibers arranged longitudinally.

The submucosa lies beneath the mucosa, provides support and contains larger blood vessels and a nerve plexus (submucosal plexus or Meissner's plexus). The glands present into the submucosa are called submucosal glands. These submucosal glands produce a mucous secretion, which lubricates the epithelium and aids the passage of food.

Muscularis externa: The submucosa is surrounded by smooth muscle, which is divided into two differently oriented layers—an inner circular and an outer longitudinal layer. Between two muscle layers is the second nerve plexus innervating the alimentary canal called myenteric plexus or Auerbach's plexus. The muscularis externa is somewhat unusual in that it contains striated muscle is its upper one-third, a mixture of striated and smooth muscle in its middle one-third and only smooth muscle in its lower one-third.

The adventitia consists of a layer of loose connective tissue, adipose tissue and neurovascular bundle.

Serosa is present only in the lower part of the esophagus (approx. the lowest 2 cm) which enters the peritoneal cavity and is lined by simple squamous epithelium (mesothelial lining).

Keys for identification: Esophagus

a. Lumen lined by mucosa consisting of stratified squamous epithelium (nonkeratinized).
b. Lamina propria is thick forming longitudinal folds.
c. Muscularis mucosa thick composed of longitudinally arranged smooth muscle fibers.

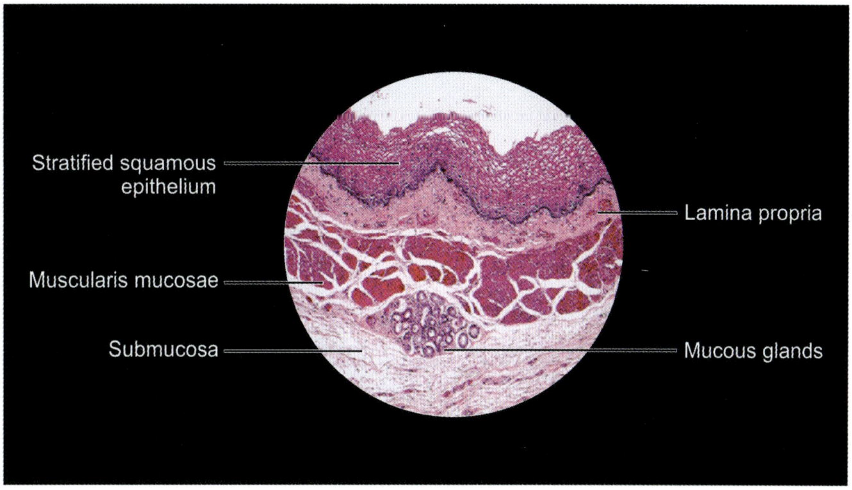

Fig. 3.20 Esophagus

Blank space for sketch work by students

STOMACH (FIGS 3.21 AND 3.22)

Functions of Stomach

- Temporary food storage
- Control the rate at which food enters the duodenum
- Acid secretion and antibacterial action
- Fluidization of stomach contents
- Preliminary digestion with pepsin, lipases, etc.

Digestion and Absorption

- Peristaltic waves occur every 20 seconds when the stomach is full
- They mix food and gastric juice in the stomach and change it to thin liquid called chyme
- Stomach pepsin is activated by stomach acid (pH 2.0) which breaks down proteins into peptides
- Mucus, secreted by mucous cells, prevents digestion of proteins in the stomach lining.

Gastric secretion and motility regulation: When chyme reaches small intestine, it releases hormones secretin and cholecystokinin.

Microanatomy

Mucosa is thrown into prominent mucosal longitudinal folds called rugosities which permit distension. It is lined by **nonciliated simple columnar epithelial cell** (mucous surface cells).

Epithelial cells go deep inside mucosal gastric pits or foveoli to form gastric glands.

Histologically there are three different zones:

1. Cardiac end—a small area of predominant mucous secreting cells.
2. Fundus and body which secrete acid peptic gastric juice and protective mucous.
3. Pylorus—the pyloric glands secrete mucous of two different types and endocrinal cells secrete gastrin.

Cell Types in the Gastric Glands

- **Surface mucous cells cover the luminal surface of stomach** and line the gastric pits. They secrete mucous and bicarbonate ions to protect the epithelium from auto digestion by gastric juice (containing HCl and pepsin) present in the stomach lumen. They have short surface microvilli.
- **Neck mucous cells** are dispersed between the parietal cells which secrete mucous that is thinner than that secreted by the surface mucous cells; mucous protects other glandular cells from action of proteases and HCl. They have large secretory granules and more polyribosomes than surface mucous cells. The mucous secreted is less alkaline than surface mucous cells.
- **Parietal (oxyntic) cells** are found throughout the gastric gland but most numerous in the isthmus; round cells that contain distinct eosinophilic (pink) cytoplasm and round, prominent nucleus; secrete HCl and intrinsic factor, needed for absorption of vitamin B_{12}. in the terminal ileum (preventing pernicious anemia).

- **Chief (peptic, zymogenic) cells** found mostly near the base of the gastric glands, very basophilic (purple) containing basal nucleus and prominent basophilic apical cytoplasm filled with many ribosomes, secrete pepsinogen, which is converted to pepsin in the acidic medium of the stomach.
- **Neuroendocrine cells** are difficult to distinguish by conventional light microscopy. Several types are present,which secrete serotonin, gastrin, glucagon, and somatostatin hormones.
- **Differentiated/Stem cells** are located primarily in the neck region difficult to identify in routine H and E sections, undergo mitosis to form more cells which differentiate into the other cell types present in the gland.

Cardiac glands are tubular slightly tortuous and occasionally branched limited to the esophageal opening. Mucosa is mainly composed of mucous secreting cells which have a basal nucleus and apical part is filled with mucin granules.

Mucosa of **fundus and body** of the stomach consists of straight tubular glands which secretes the gastric juice. Gastric juice is the mixture of mucous, HCl and pepsinogen.

The pits occupy only ¼ of mucosa and has 1–7 glands opening into it, each gland has a mouth opening in the pit, a short isthmus containing dividing cells and undifferentiated cells, a constricted portion the neck containing neck mucous cells, parietal cells and enteroendocrinal cells.

The body and slightly dilated and folded blind end is fundus which contains chief cells, some parietal cells and several types of enteroendocrinal cells. Mucosa is secretory not absorptive but some water, salts, lipid soluble drugs, alcohol and aspirin may enter lamina propria by damaging the surface epithelium.

Pyloric region: Pyloric glands of gastric mucosa are located in the pyloric antrum, lumen is wider, secretory cells are similar to surface mucous cells but the secretion is more viscid, enteroendocrinal, few parietal cells are also present. The gastric pits into which glands empty are much deeper and occupy half the thickness of mucosa.

Lamina propria packed with gastric glands, reticular fibers, fibroblasts, plasma cells, macrophages, blood vessels, nerves and small lymphatic nodules.

Muscularis mucosae has inner circular and outer longitudinal muscle fibers and in few cases an outer third circular layer may be present. Thin strands of smooth muscles may extend in the lamina propria to help in outflow of gastric glands secretions.

Sub mucosa consists of loose connective tissue that contains fat, blood vessels and Meissner's plexus which innervates the blood vessels of submucosa and smooth muscles of muscularis mucosae.

Muscularis externa: Stomach has three smooth muscle layers:

1. Oblique inner layer
2. Circular middle layer
3. Longitudinal outer layer.

It has parasympathetic myenteric (Auerbach's plexus) orientation of these smooth muscles is exactly not in layers but in a random manner, i.e. in a way that mixes the chyme during digestion as well as its ability to force the partially digested food into the small intestine.

Serosa: The serous coat consists of a layer of loosely arranged connective tissue which is covered by mesothelium.

Keys for identification: Fundic part and body

a. Mucosa thrown into folds, lined by columnar epithelium with no villi and no goblet cells.
b. Gastric pits extend up to 1/4 thickness of the mucosa.
c. Parietal cells seen.

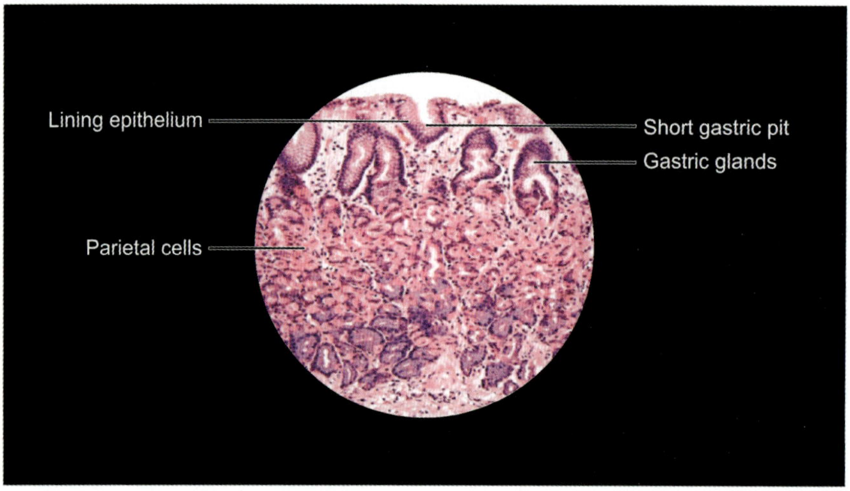

Fig. 3.21 Stomach (Fundus)

Blank space for sketch work by students

Keys for identification: Pyloric part

a. Mucosa thrown into folds, lined by columnar epithelium with no villi and no goblet cells.
b. Gastric pits extend up to 1/2 of the thickness of the mucosa.
c. Light stained mucoid cells seen.

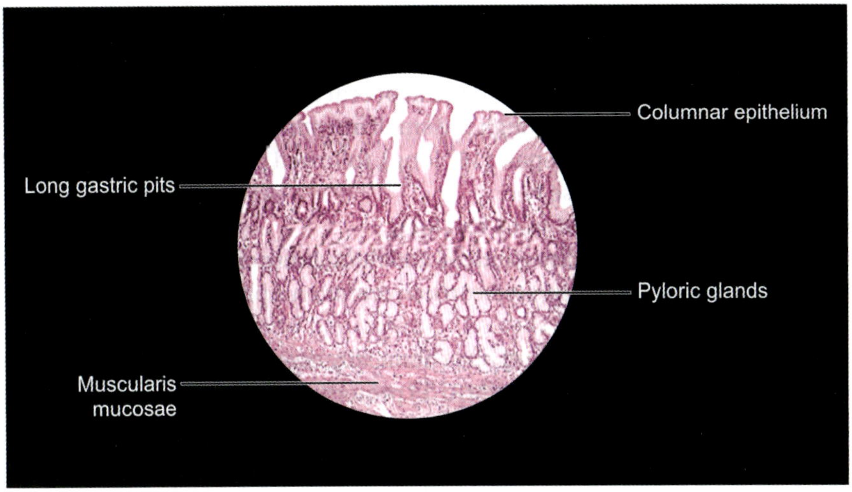

Fig. 3.22 Stomach (Pyloric)

Blank space for sketch work by students

macrophages and fenestrated capillaries and a central blind ending lymph capillary called lacteal and smooth muscles derived from muscularis mucosae that contracts and forces the lymph into the lymph vessels.

- Individual cells have numerous projections of their apical plasma membranes called **microvilli** which are microscopic projections on absorptive cells (200 million/mm^2).
- The mucosa and submucosa together form large transverse folds into the lumen called **plicae circulares**—permanent ridges in mucosa that cause chyme to spiral.
- The small intestine is extremely long (usually several meters).

DUODENUM (FIGS 3.23 TO 3.25)

Mucosa is thrown into finger like processes called **villi** covered by **simple columnar epithelium** with a brush border. Villi are short, numerous, shaped like a leaf and closely packed.

Between the villi are intestinal glands which extend up to the muscularis mucosae.

Lamina propria: No lymphocytic aggregations are seen.

Below **muscularis mucosae** is **submucosa** which is filled by a large number of mucous glands called **Brunner's glands** which deliver their secretory products into the bases of intestinal glands. Presence of chyme in the small intestine induces cells of Brunner's glands to secrete alkaline mucus that neutralizes gastric acid and pepsin and further promotes digestion.

Surrounding this is **muscularis externa** which consists of inner circular and outer longitudinal layer of smooth muscles.

Serosa is a fibrous layer covered with mesothelium.

Keys for identification: Duodenum

a. Presence of Brunner's glands in the submucosa.
b. No plicae circulares.
c. Longest villi of all three regions.
d. Highest number of goblet cells.

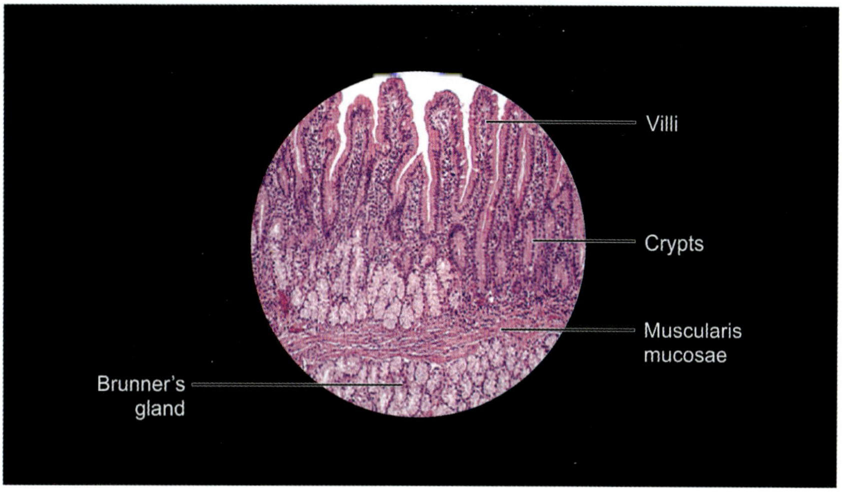

Fig. 3.23 Duodenum Brunner's glands

Blank space for sketch work by students

Keys for identification: Jejunum

a. Simple columnar epithelium with tall villi and goblet cells.
b. Absence of Brunner' s gland in submucosa.
c. Absence of Peyer's patches in submucosa.

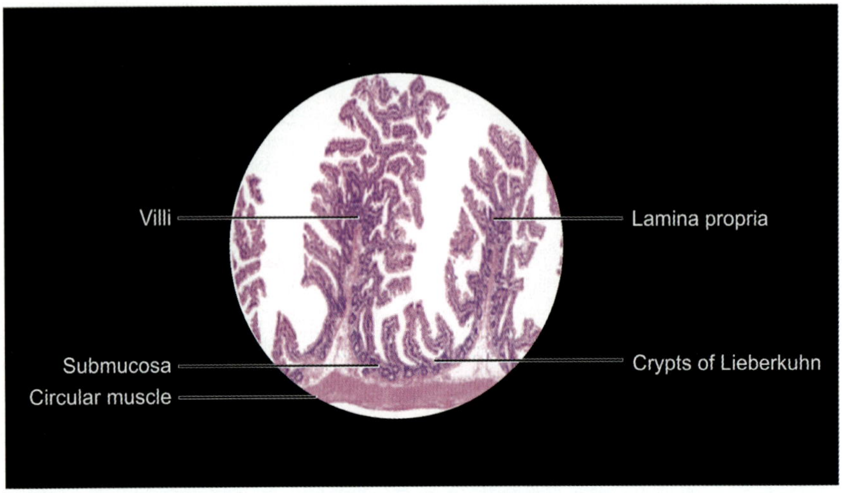

Fig. 3.24 Jejunum

Blank space for sketch work by students

Keys for identification: Ileum

a. Permanent aggregated lymphoid nodules in the submucosa (Peyer's patches).
b. Shortest villi.
c. Least number of goblet cells.

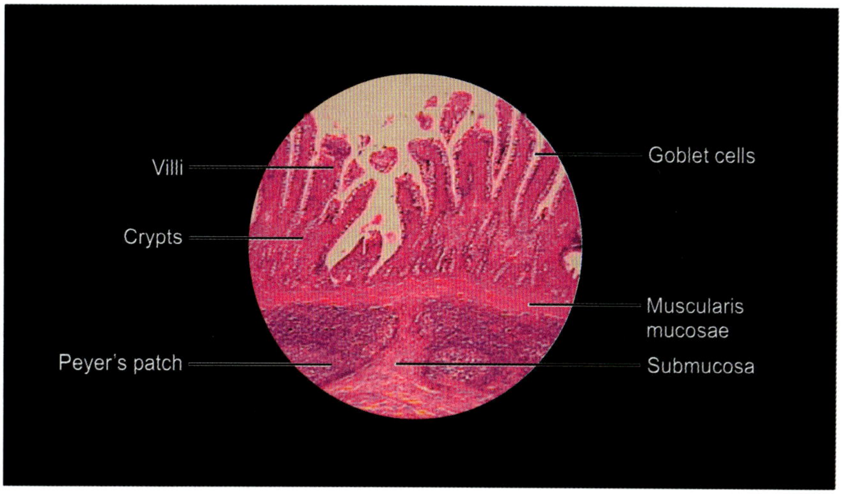

Fig. 3.25 Ileum

Blank space for sketch work by students

APPENDIX (FIG. 3.26)

- It is the narrowest part of gut and blind ended tubular organ.
- Site for digestion of cellulose by symbiotic bacteria in herbivores.

Microanatomy

Mucosa: Lined by **columnar epithelium**, also contains follicle associated epithelial cells (FAE cells) or M cells or microfold cells. They are modified enterocytes that cover enlarged lymphatic nodules in the lamina propria which is involved in sampling of antigens in the lumen of appendix.

Crypts are few and less closely packed than anywhere else in large gut.

Lamina propria is rich in lymphoid tissue and extends into submucosa. Lymphoid follicles with germinal centers are seen (GALT).

Submucosa is well developed with lymphoid masses.

Muscularis externa is composed of a thick inner layer of circular and thin layer of outer longitudinal smooth muscle coat.

Serosa forms a complete covering by the mesothelial cells and submesothelial connective tissue.

Keys for identification: Appendix

a. Lumen small.
b. Lamina propria and submucosa diffusely infiltrated with lymphoid tissue.
c. Mucosal glands are much less closely packed.

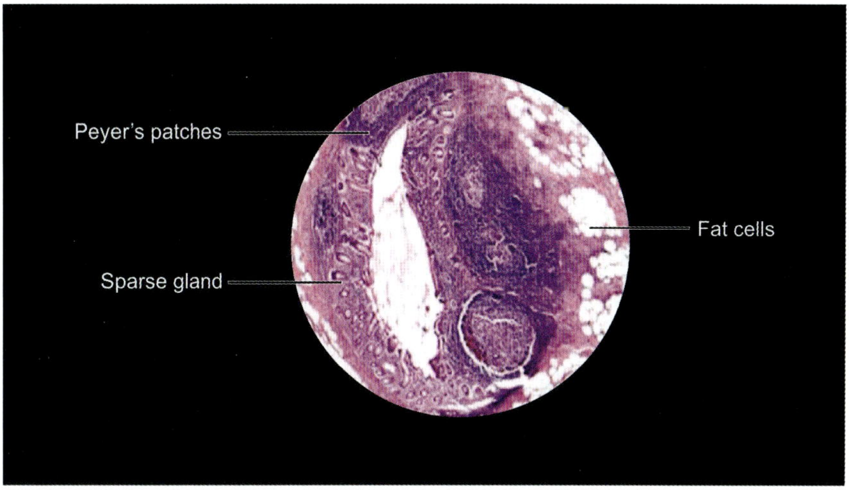

Fig. 3.26 Appendix

Blank space for sketch work by students

COLON (FIG. 3.27)

The principal function of large gut is reabsorption of water, electrolytes and vitamins and excretion of undigested food and wastes. Commensal bacteria reside in the large intestine and further degrade food residue. Small quantities of fat soluble vitamins derived from bacterial activity are absorbed in large gut. Intraepithelial lymphocytes, plasma cells and lymphocytes in lamina propria and lymphoid aggregates in lamina propria and submucosa form the defence mechanisms against invading organisms.

Microanatomy

Mucosa is folded but distinct plica circulares are not present, only temporary folds are there.

Epithelium

There are **no villi** so the surface of the mucosa is smooth and flatter than that of small intestine.

The lining epithelium is **simple columnar** that forms straight long tubular glands (**crypts of Lieberkuhn**) which are deeper, more in number than in small intestine, extend up to the muscularis mucosae and are separated by thin plates of lamina propria. These glands are lined with absorptive columnar cells similar to enterocytes of small intestine (which recover water and salts) and numerous goblet cells producing mucus to facilitate the passage of dry waste material.

The lining epithelium also contains **stem cells** located at the bottom of intestinal gland causing renewal of absorptive and **goblet cells** (6 days), **enteroendocrinal cells** (4 weeks) and intraepithelial lymphocytes. There are no **Paneth cells**.

Lamina propria is **thick, crypts** are **longer and densely packed**, consists of loose connective tissue that contains numerous blood and lymphatic vessels, collagen, lymphocytes and plasma cells.

Muscularis mucosae present beneath the base of the crypts and prominent identifying feature. It is arranged in two layers inner circular and outer longitudinal which undergo rhythmic contractions. It is traversed by diffuse lymphoid tissue which extend from lamina propria to submucosa.

Submucosa: is typical consisting of connective tissue, nerves and blood vessels.

Muscularis externa consists of inner circular and outer longitudinal layers which is thickened and organized into three separate bands known as *Taenia coli* (except for rectum, anal canal and appendix).

Serosa is usual and fat filled pouches known as appendices epiploicae are seen. Parts of the colon which have no serosa are covered with adventitia.

Keys for identification: Colon

a. No villi so the surface is flat and smooth.
b. Goblet cells in abundance.
c. Presence of *Taenia coli*.

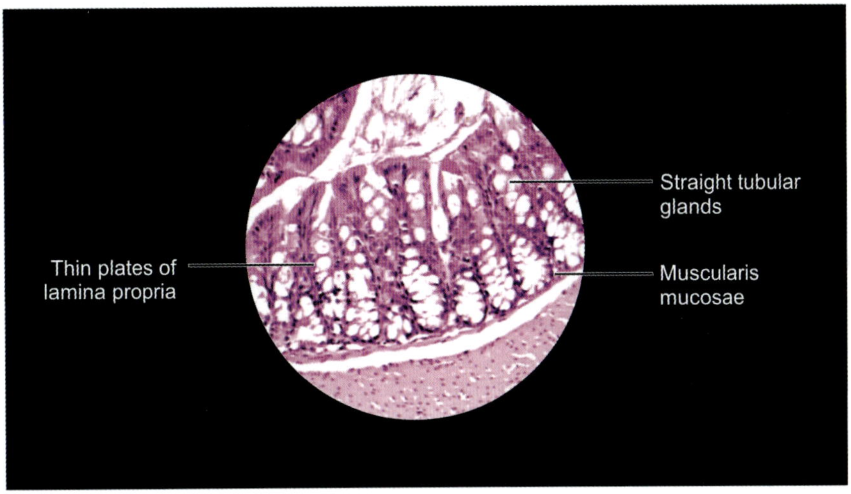

Fig. 3.27 Colon

Blank space for sketch work by students

LIVER (FIG. 3.28)

- The liver is the second largest organ in the body (next to skin).
- It is an endocrine as well as an exocrine gland.

Exocrine Functions

Synthesis and release of bile, emulsifies fat that is digested by pancreatic amylase and absorbed in the intestines by lacteals.

Endocrine Functions

- Secretions of liver include albumin, globulins prothrombin, glycoproteins, glucose released from stored glycogen and tri-iodothyronine is directly released into the blood.
- Liver consists of functional units called **hepatic lobules** with a central vein in the center and portal triads at the periphery.
- **Portal lobule** is a triangular block of tissue with portal triad at the center and central vein at the periphery. This emphasizes exocrine function of liver, i.e. these lobules secrete bile which drains into the axial bile duct.
- **Liver acinus** provides the best correlation between the perfusion of blood, metabolic activity and liver pathology. In this the long axis passes through central veins and short axis between portal triads and thus divides into three zones.
  - Zone 1 receives most oxygenated blood which is rich in nutrients also.
  - Zone 2 transition zone.
  - Zone 3 is first to show ischemic changes and fat accumulation and last to respond to toxic changes and bile stasis.

Microanatomy

- It is covered by a dense fibroelastic capsule known as Glisson's capsule.
- The classical hepatic lobule is between central vein and the peripheral connective tissue of interlobular septum (3–6 portal triads). Plates of hepatic cells (usually one cell thick) radiate from the central vein towards the periphery. **Hepatocytes** are large polyhedral cells which have 6 or more surfaces with large spherical nucleus and eosinophilic cytoplasm. More than half of the hepatocytes contain twice the amount of normal (diploid) amount of chromosome in a single nucleus, i.e. they are tetraploid and some contain 4–8 times of this amount (polypoidy). Some cells are binucleate.
- Branches of portal vein and hepatic artery penetrate the septum and form sinusoids between plates of hepatic cells.
- These sinusoids are lined by three types of cells:
  1. **Discontinuous endothelial cells** and do not have a basement membrane. All the sinusoids drain towards and open in central vein.
  2. Sinusoids also contain phagocytic **Kupffer's cells** (part of MPS) which are large cells with several processes, irregular/stellate in outline and protrude into the sinusoids. Kupffer's cells in the sinusoids destroy pathogens and worn out blood cells. The nuclei are obscured by the ingested materials.

3. **Ito cells** (stellate cells or hepatic lipocytes) are present in the perisinusoidal space and have small lipid droplets containing vitamin A in the cytoplasm thus having a dual function of vitamin A storage and production of extracellular matrix and collagen. During liver injury these cells are thought to produce increased amounts of collagen causing the fibrosis which is characteristic of liver cirrhosis.

- A narrow space (**space of Disse**) separates the sinusoids from the hepatocytes (perisinusoidal space) which drain into the lymphatics of portal tracts.
- There are minute canaliculi formed by opposing surfaces of hepatocytes, near the portal canal. They merge to form **Herring canals** whose characteristics feature is that it is lined by both hepatocytes and cholangiocytes.
- **Space of Mall** is a small space between outermost hepatocyte and the edges of portal canal. This space is thought to be one of the sites where lymph originates in liver.

Blood Supply to the Liver

In a classic hepatic lobule, hepatocytes (liver cells) are arranged radially around a central vein. With 3-6 portal triads at the periphery each consisting of a branch of hepatic artery bile duct and portal vein (largest).

Liver is unusual in having both arterial and venous blood supplies, oxygen through hepatic artery and nutrient rich blood from portal vein. The venous drainage is through hepatic veins into the inferior vena cava.

Blood then flows into liver sinusoids where:

- Hepatocytes take up oxygen, nutrients and toxins and remove wastes (CO_2).
- Kupffer's cells remove dead matter and pathogens.

Sinusoids drain blood into central vein → hepatic vein → inferior vena cava → Right atrium.

Keys for identification: Liver

a. Hepatocytes arranged radially around central vein seen.
b. Presence of portal triad at the periphery.
c. Hepatic sinusoids lined by Kupffer's cells seen.

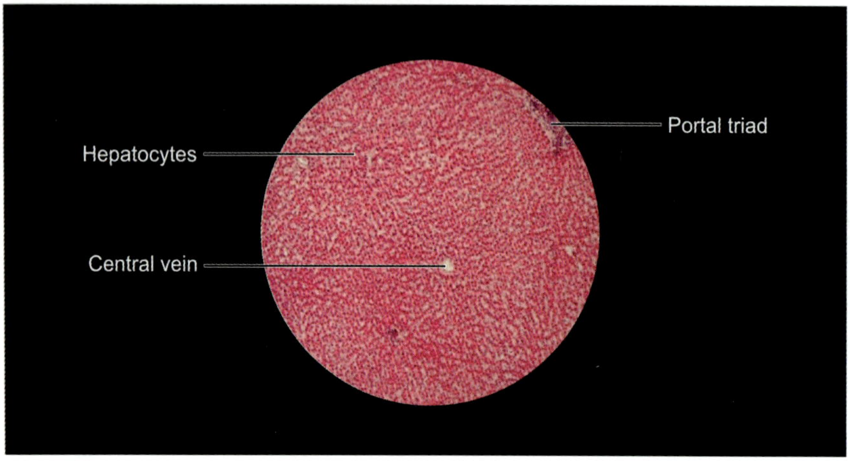

Fig. 3.28 Liver

Blank space for sketch work by students

GALLBLADDER (FIG. 3.29)

The gallbladder concentrates and stores bile that is produced in the liver.

Microanatomy

Mucosa is characterized by tall columnar absorptive cells, the cytoplasm is stained uniformly and intercellular spaces at their bases are distended. One cell type epithelium with numerous short apical processes (brush border) with oval basal nuclei is seen. In contracted state mucosa in thrown into folds (like villi) the recess in between the folds resembles a gland. But this epithelial lined structure is not a true gland, it is an invagination of mucosa extending into or through the thickness of muscularis externa. These invaginations are called as Rokitansky Aschoff sinuses. Villi and glands are absent except a few glands are present in the fundus.

Lamina propria is highly cellular.

Muscularis mucosae is absent.

Muscularis externa consists of interlacing bundles of smooth muscles.

Adventitia consists of irregular dense connective tissues along with blood vessels and adipose tissue at the periphery.

Keys for identification: Gallbladder

a. Tall columnar epithelium with brush border thrown into folds.
b. But there are no villi and no glands.
c. No goblet cells and no muscularis mucosae.

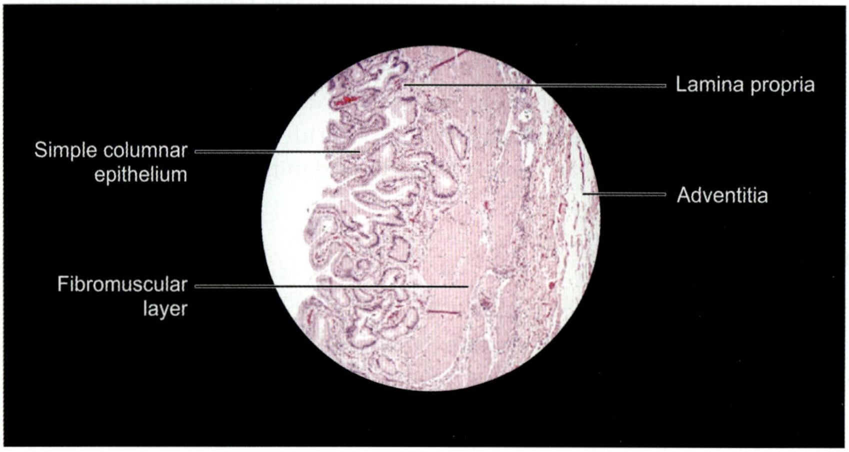

Fig. 3.29 Gallbladder

Blank space for sketch work by students

PANCREAS (FIG. 3.30)

- The pancreas is both an endocrine and exocrine gland.
- The pancreas produces the hormones insulin and glucagon directly into the bloodstream (endocrine function).
- It is a **compound tubuloacinar** type of gland, produces pancreatic juice rich in enzymes which plays an important role in the chemical digestion of food (**exocrine function**).
- Pancreatic secretions reach duodenum via the pancreatic duct (unites with the common bile duct).
- Ninety-nine percent of pancreatic cells are arranged in clusters called acini (secrete pancreatic juice).
- One percent of pancreatic cells, **Islets of Langerhans**, secrete hormones—insulin, glucagon, somatostatin and pancreatic polypeptide.
- In response to acidic chyme in the small intestine secretin secreted by enteroendocrinal cells stimulates the centroacinar cells and cells lining the intercalated ducts to secrete large amounts of watery fluid rich in bicarbonate ions to neutralize the acidic chyme.
- In response to presence of fats and proteins in the small intestine, cholecystokinin release stimulates acinar cells to secrete digestive enzymes which enter the duodenum in an inactive form which are activated by hormones secreted by intestinal mucosa.

Microanatomy

Exocrine Part

- There is a capsule made up of thin collagen fibers which extend as fibrous septas between the lobules.
- A large number of closely packed serous acini arranged into lobules, composed of large darkly stained cells drained by intralobular ducts which drain into larger interlobular ducts.
- The cells of the serous acini are roughly truncated pyramidal in shape, basophilic with apical portion filled with eosinophilic granules, nucleus is rounded and located at the base.
- The epithelium of **intercalated duct** is **low cuboidal** which penetrates partially into the acini (so the lumen is small in size) forming the pale staining **centroacinar cells**.
- The intercalated ducts secrete water and bicarbonate ions into the pancreatic juice. There are no striated **ducts**.
- **Intercalated ducts** drain into **intralobular ducts** which in turn drain into **interlobular ducts**. The epithelium becomes stratified cuboidal in larger ducts.
- The main pancreatic duct is covered by a thick layer of dense connective tissue and may contain smooth muscles.

Endocrine Part

- The **islets of Langerhans** are larger in area than the **acini**.
- It is seen as group of pale staining spherical cells separated by fine collagen fibers containing fenestrated capillaries and surrounded by a thin layer of reticular fibers.

- Differentiated from parotid by:
  1. Presence of islets of Langerhans.
  2. Centroacinar cells.
  3. Absence of striated ducts.
  4. No lobes only lobules and less connective tissue but serous acini are common.

Keys for identification: Pancreas (Exocrine)

a. Composed of serous acini.
b. Centroacinar cells seen.
c. No strated ducts.

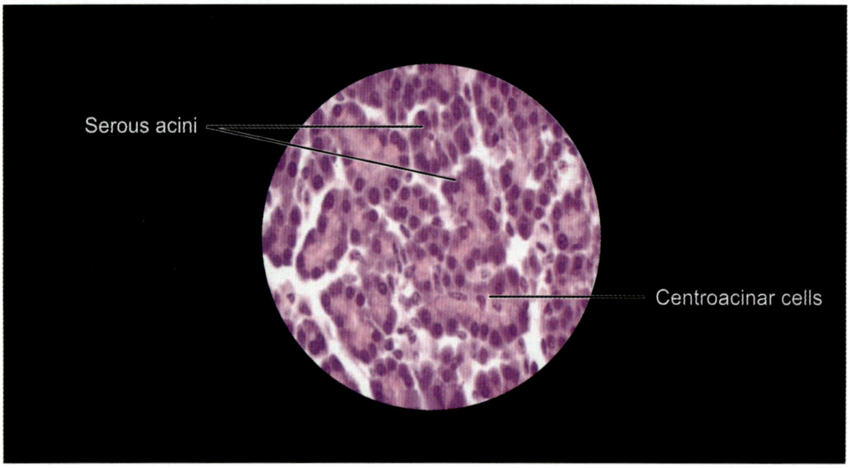

Fig. 3.30 Pancreas (Exocrine)

Blank space for sketch work by students

URINARY SYSTEM

The kidneys, ureters, urinary bladder and urethra are the main components of the urinary system. The functions of the urinary system are:

1. Controls the water and electrolyte balance in the body.
2. Helps to regulate the blood pressure by renin-angiotensin-aldosterone mechanism.
3. Excretion of many toxic metabolites like urea, nitrogen and creatinine.
4. Maintenance of acid base balance.
5. Also functions as an endocrine organ by the release of hormone erythropoietin, which stimulates the formation of red blood cells in the bone marrow.

The kidney consists of **cortex, medulla** and the **pelvis**. The segments of cortex and pyramid (in the medulla) form a **renal lobe** (10–18 lobes). Medullary ray and surrounding cortical tissue form **renal lobule**.

The **cortex** consists of the **renal corpuscles** which appear as dense rounded mass formed by a bunch of capillaries (glomerulus) lying in two layered cup known as Bowman's capsule and **convoluted tubules, junctional tubules and thick segments of loop of Henle**.

The **medulla** consists of a number of **renal pyramids** having thin segments of **loops of Henle, collecting tubules and collecting ducts**.

The cortex and medulla drain into the pelvis which is the hollow and funnel shaped beginning of the **ureter**. The renal **calyces, the pelvis and ureters** are lined by **transitional epithelium**.

The kidney is made up of large numbers of **uriniferous** tubules which consist of **nephrons** (about 1–2 millions) and the **collecting tubules**. Nephrons are the basic functional unit of the kidney. It is comprised of renal corpuscle (**Malpighian corpuscle**), i.e. the glomerulus and renal tubule which includes Bowman's capsule, **proximal convoluted tubule, loop of Henle and distal convoluted tubule**. Filtration is done by the glomeruli of the kidney whereas selective reabsorption is performed by the tubular system of the kidney. The interlobular arteries extend numerous afferent glomerular arteries to the glomeruli. The diameter of **afferent arteriole** is more than **efferent arteriole** so a pressure gradient is created which causes active filtration of components of blood into the Bowman's space as glomerular filtrate.

CORTICAL NEPHRONS

- Located in the cortex.
- Have short loops of Henle that extend only up to outer medulla.

Juxtamedullary Nephrons are 1/7th of total nephrons.

- Located at the corticomedullary junction.
- They have long loops of Henle that extend deep into the medulla accompanied by vasa recta.
- They produce a hypertonic environment in the interstitium of medulla necessary for the production of hypertonic urine.

Types of Cells in the Glomerulus

1. Endothelial cells.
2. Podocytes.
3. Mesangial cells.

The **glomerulus** is enclosed by two layers of **Bowman's capsule**. Cells of the outer or parietal layer of Bowman's capsule form a simple squamous epthelium. Cells of the inner layer consist of podocytes in the visceral layer which surrounds the glomerular capillaries and are extremely complex in shape. They give rise to thin long cytoplasmic primary processes which further form secondary processes (**pedicels**) that surround the capillaries and interdigitate with secondary processes of other podocytes. The cell bodies of podocytes and their primary processes do not touch glomerular basement membranes. The gaps between these interdigitations are called **slit pores** or **filtration slits bridged** by **slit membrane**. A thick basement membrane is formed by the fusion of basal lamina of endothelial cells and podocytes so during filtration the glomerular filtrate passes through the fenestrated endothelium of glomerular capillary (acts as coarse filter), glomerular basement membrane and slit membranes then filtration slits between secondary processes of podocytes. Both kidneys produce 125 mL of filtrate per minute out of which 124 mL is reabsorbed and only 1 mL per minute is excreted into the renal pelvis (total urine formed per day is 1500 mL).

Mesangial cells in the glomerulus form the connective tissue that gives structural support to podocytes and vessels.

Renal **tubules** are long folded structures. It is up to 55 mm long in humans and extends from Bowman's capsule to its junction with a collecting tubule.

The renal tubules receive filtrate from the **glomerulus** and process it into urine.

Each tubule is differentiated into several specialized segments.

Different aspects of filtrate reabsorption are localized in different segments.

- The **proximal tubules** in the cortex, reabsorb most minerals and other nutrients from the tubular fluid and passes them to blood in the **peritubular capillaries**.

  The **loop of Henle** dips into the **medulla** where it helps to establish the hypertonic environment of medullary interstitial fluid.
- The **distal convoluted tubule** returns to the **juxtaglomerular apparatus** of the corpuscle from which the tubule arose.
- Finally, the collecting duct leads back through the medulla to drain into the renal pelvis.

PROXIMAL CONVOLUTED TUBULE

It is called proximal because it is nearest to the renal corpuscle and **convoluted** because it twists about.

It restores much of the filtrate to the blood in the **peritubular capillaries** by actively pumping small molecules out of the tubular lumen into the interstitial space. Water then follows the concentration gradient.

It is the initial segment of the renal tubule, 50–60 microns in diameter characterized by **eosinophilic, low columnar cells/large cuboidal cells**. The apical end of each cell has a **brush border of microvilli**. This provides an increased surface area to accommodate the membrane channels that are responsible for absorbing into the cell small molecules from the filtrate in the tubular lumen. The brush border is not always seen and the lumen is filled with a fuzzy material which represents the remaining of the brush border of the cells as it is not well preserved in the section. Proximal tubule cells have indistinct apical ends. The length of a proximal convoluted tubule tends to be several times greater than that of **a distal convoluted tubule**, so sections seen are of proximal tubules than those of distal tubules. The cells have a high proportion of mitochondria in their cytoplasm, to provide the energy for pumping ions and molecules against their concentration gradient. The abundance of mitochondria makes the cells intensely **acidophilic**.

The plasma membranes of adjacent proximal tubule cells are extensively interdigitated. This increases the basal membrane surface area available for pumping molecules out of the basal end of each cell. As a consequence of such interdigitated cell membranes, boundaries between adjacent proximal convoluted tubule cells are not clear (i.e. the epithelium looks like a continuous band of cytoplasm with nuclei appearing at irregular intervals).

The epithelium of the initial thick descending segment of the **loop of Henle** is similar to that of the proximal convoluted tubule, and is sometimes called the **pars recta** then is, **thin descending limb, thin ascending limb, thick ascending limb** leading into the **straight part of the distal tubule**, which is formed by low cuboidal cells without a brush border. A few short microvilli are present, but they are difficult to see in the light microscope. The diameter of the tubule expands to 35 mm. Epithelial cells in the ascending parts of the intermediate and straight distal tubule cells transport chloride (active) and sodium ions (passive) out of the tubular lumen into the surrounding peritubular space. The epithelium is impermeable to water. Consequently, the transport of ions over the epithelium sets up a gradient in osmotic pressure, which serves as driving force in the further concentration of the urine.

DISTAL CONVOLUTED TUBULE

They are 20–50 microns in diameter. Like the proximal convoluted tubule, it is called **convoluted** because it twists about and is called **distal** because it is further away from the renal corpuscle. They can be distinguished from the proximal tubules by the **smaller size**, a much larger lumen, lined by cuboidal cells which **do not have a brush border** and they **stain less lightly** than proximal tubules. Sections of distal convoluted tubules tend to be less in number, because distal tubules are much shorter and less convoluted than proximal tubules. The distal convoluted tubule continues into the cortex from the ascending thick limb of the **loop of Henle**. This segment of the renal tubule continues the return of useful materials from the filtrate to the blood in the **peritubular capillaries**, like the proximal convoluted tubule by actively pumping small molecules out of the tubular lumen into the interstitial space.

JUXTAGLOMERULAR APPARATUS

Each distal tubule returns to the **vascular pole** of the **renal corpuscle** from which the tubule arose. At this site is a special region called **juxtaglomerular (JG) apparatus**. The juxtaglomerular apparatus is a complex of structures associated with the vascular pole of each renal corpuscle and is thought to participate in the regulation of blood flow through the glomerular capillaries (and hence the rate of urine formation). JG apparatus maintains the normal blood pressure and it consist of juxtaglomerular cells in the walls of afferent arteriole. These are specialized smooth muscle cells containing granules secreting renin. JG cells produce and secrete renin. Renin activates angiotensinogen, a precursor found in the bloodstream, leading to the formation of angiotensin I that is converted to angiotensin II by a converting enzyme in the lungs. Angiotensin II is the most potent vasoconstrictor known. Angiotensin II also stimulates the secretion of aldosterone from the adrenal cortex which acts on the cells of distal convoluted tubules to increase reabsorption of sodium and chloride ions from the glomerular filtrate so water follows osmotically increasing the fluid volume thus raising the blood pressure.

Macula densa is an area of densely packed nuclei of epithelial cells of distal convoluted tubule adjacent to the afferent arteriole at the vascular pole of corpuscle. It functions as a sensor for sodium/or chloride concentration. The straight portion of the distal tubule contacts the glomerulus forming the macula densa. Thereafter, the distal tubule forms its convoluted portion (about 5 mm long). Cells in the distal tubules are sensitive to the hormone aldosterone, which is produced in the zona glomerulosa of the adrenal glands. Aldosterone stimulates the active resorption of sodium ions and the excretion of potassium ions.

Lacis cells also called extraglomerular mesangial cells or Goormaghtigh cells. They form a conical mass between afferent and efferent arterioles and macula densa. They provide support and transmit the signals arising in the macula densa to intraglomerular mesangial cells which contract or relax the capillary loops to maintain blood pressure.

Glomerular filtrate flows from distal convoluted tubule to the collecting tubule which is not a part of nephron.

THE COLLECTING TUBULES

They join to form the larger straight collecting ducts known as papillary ducts or the Ducts of Bellini which empty into the minor calyx at the summit of renal papilla.

Collecting tubules have a **large lumen** which is **circular** in contrast to the **irregular shapes of convoluted tubules**, consisting of **principal and intercalated** cells.

COLLECTING DUCTS

The convoluted distal tubules merge, via connecting or junctional tubules, with the collecting ducts. They are easily recognized in the renal medulla. They are so named because they "collect" the urine from distal convoluted tubules. Collecting ducts are lined by simple cuboidal epithelium which appears less specialized than that of the proximal or distal tubules. The cytoplasm is relatively clear (i.e. not intensely eosinophilic) and cell borders are usually distinct. Collecting ducts merge and become larger as they descend through the medulla, so different sizes of collecting ducts may be observed at different levels in the kidney, with the smallest in the cortex and the largest near the pelvis. Collecting ducts merge to form papillary ducts of Bellini, which terminate on the tips of the renal papilla and empty into a distended, funnel shaped part (minor calyx) of the ureter. In the presence of antidiuretic hormone (ADH), the epithelia of the collecting ducts are permeable to water but not to sodium ions. Osmotic forces move water out of the lumen of the tubules as they pass through the medulla, where cells of the ascending intermediate and straight distal tubules of the loop of Henle have established high concentrations of sodium in the extracellular space.

When there is dehydration or decreased water intake in the body ADH (acts on collecting tubules and collecting ducts) is secreted from the posterior pituitary and water is reabsorbed from the filtrate (due to increased permeability and the osmotic pressure created by hypertonic extracellular fluid through counter-current multiplier system) into the interstitium from where it is returned to general circulation via vasa recta, the filtrate in collecting tubules becomes hypertonic (concentrated) so ADH causes water retention and production of hypertonic urine. Conversely, ADH secretion is inhibited by water overload and an increased volume of hypertonic urine is produced. Collecting tubules and collecting ducts are sites for H^+ ion secretion and thus important for acid-base balance.

VASCULAR SUPPLY

It is by the renal artery which divides into segmental branches. These branches further divide into interlobar arteries, arcuate arteries, interlobular arteries and afferent arterioles which supply blood to the glomerular capillaries which are drained by efferent arterioles. These form a peritubular capillary plexus around the convoluted tubules in the cortical nephrons. In juxtamedullary nephrons they form long thin vasa recta (necessary for the production of concentrated urine) and ultimately drain into the renal vein.

Microanatomy (Figs 3.31 and 3.32)

The kidney consists of outer perirenal fat, connective tissue capsule, cortex and medulla.

The cortex consists of the renal corpuscles which appears as dense rounded mass formed by a bundles of capillaries (glomerulus) lying in two layered cup known as Bowman's capsule and convoluted tubules junctional tubules and thick segments of loop of Henle. The medullary rays do not extend up to the capsule because of a narrow zone of convoluted tubules.

The proximal convoluted tubules make up most of cortex. The length of a proximal convoluted tubule tends to be several times greater than that of a distal convoluted tubule, so sections seen are mostly of proximal tubules than distal tubules. It is **eosinophilic** due to large number of mitochondria, lined by large cuboidal cells having **a brush border of microvilli**. The brush border is not always seen as the lumen is filled with a fuzzy material which represents the remaining of the brush border which is not well preserved in the section. Apical ends are not distinct. The epithelium looks like a continuous band of cytoplasm with nuclei appearing at irregular intervals.

Distal convoluted tubules: can be distinguished from the proximal tubules by the **smaller size, lined by cuboidal cells** which do not have a brush border **so lumen** appears **larger** and they stain less lightly than proximal tubules. Sections of distal convoluted tubules tend to be less in number, because distal tubules are much shorter in length.

Medulla comprises renal pyramids whose apex is directed inwards forming the papilla which projects into the minor calyx. It contains only thick straight portions of descending proximal tubules, loops of Henle (thin segment). Thick ascending distal tubules, collecting tubules descend in the medulla to form collecting ducts.

The **thick descending and ascending** parts are having same features as their convoluted portions lined by **simple cuboidal epithelium with no brush border**.

Loop of Henle is the continuation of proximal convoluted tubule in cortex. It dips into the medulla as descending limb and an ascending limb which is continuous with distal convoluted tubule at the corticomedullary junction. The descending limb has a short thick segment which is the straight part of proximal convoluted tubule and a long thin segment. The ascending limb has a short thin segment and a long thick segment which is the straight part of distal convoluted tubule.

The **thin segments of loop of Henle** are lined by **simple squamous epithelium** but differentiated from capillaries by slightly larger regular, round lumen and absence of RBCs.

Vasa recta (blood vessels) are lined by **endothelial cells** which are simple squamous cells and differentiated from thin segments of loop of Henle by the presence of blood.

Collecting tubules or junctional tubules join distal convoluted tubules with **collecting ducts,** descend in the medullary ray and towards the renal medulla where they merge to form the larger **Ducts of Bellini** which drain into the renal papilla.

Smaller collecting tubules are lined by simple cuboidal epithelium, larger tubules by simple columnar and ducts of Bellini by tall columnar cells, which consists of two cell types, **principal cells and intercalated cells**. The principal cells have pale cytoplasm, luminal microvilli, cilium and contains prominent basal infoldings but no lateral interdigitations. These cells actively reabsorb Na and H_2O and secrete K^+. Intercalated cells have darker cytoplasm due to many mitochondria and their function is to secrete H^+, reabsorb HCO_3 and thus maintain acid-base balance of body.

Keys for identification: Kidney (Cortex)

a. It consists of cortex, medulla and pelvis.
b. Cortex consists of glomeruli, proximal and distal convoluted tubules.
c. Medulla contains straight portions of tubules, loops of Henle, collecting tubules and collecting ducts.

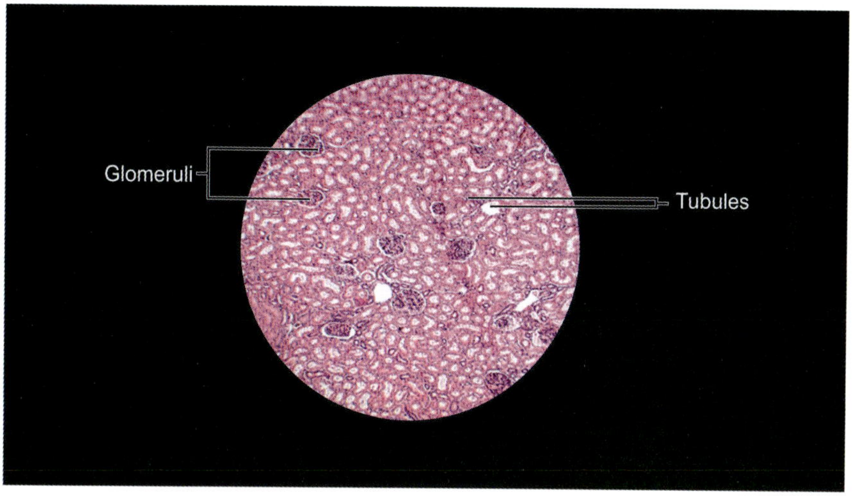

Fig. 3.31 Kidney (Cortex)

Blank space for sketch work by students

Keys for identification: Kidney

a. It consists of cortex, medulla and pelvis.
b. Cortex consists of glomeruli, proximal and distal convoluted tubules.
c. Medulla contains straight portions of tubules, loops of Henle, collecting tubules and collecting ducts.

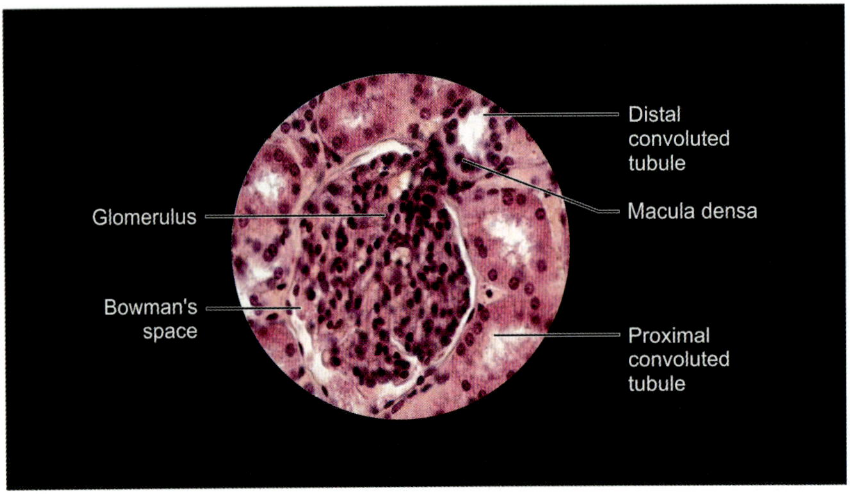

Fig. 3.32 Kidney

Blank space for sketch work by students

EXCRETORY PASSAGES

The minor calyces join to form **major calyces** within the kidney, which in turn merge to form the **renal pelvis** (still within the kidney). The urine flows through these structures to the ureter and then reaches the bladder.

The basic structure of all these components is the same.

The mucosa is lined by a transitional epithelium, seen exclusively in the urinary system, also called urothelium which lines the calyces, renal pelvis, ureter, bladder and the initial portion of prostatic urethra up to the opening of ejaculatory duct. The epithelium is impenetrable to any components of the urine, which does not change in composition as it passes through the excretory passages.

The transitional epithelium is stratified consisting of 3-6 layers. The number of layers is more when the organ is relaxed. The cells of the basal layer are cuboidal or columnar, intermediate cells are polygonal and surface cells are called umbrella cells which have unique features making this epithelium impervious to the effects of urine even when it is fully distended. The surface membrane called cuticle or glycocalyx is seen as a thin eosinophilic band which makes the cell impermeable to urine. Secondly, this impermeable barrier also prevents the water being drawn through the epithelium into the hypertonic urine. The umbrella cells are large and ovoid with round nuclei having eosinophilic cytoplasm. In some of the cells, the nuclei are in binucleate to octanucleate form. The thickened areas in the plasma membrane are called plaques which invaginate into the cell and appear as if they are folded inwards upon themselves and appear as fusiform vesicles but their lumen is in continuity with cell's exterior. Filaments attach to the undersurface of plaques which prevent undue stretching of distended bladder. The basal cells are the smallest and nuclei appear crowded because of minimal cytoplasm in each cell.

The lamina propria consists mainly of dense connective tissue, with many bundles of coarse collagenous fibers.

The muscularis externa usually consists of an inner longitudinal and outer circular layer of smooth muscle fibers. In lower parts of the ureter and the bladder, an additional outer longitudinal layer of muscles is added to the first two.

THE URETERS (FIG. 3.33)

They are the muscular tubes which carry the urine from the kidney to the bladder which is propelled by the peristaltic action of ureteric wall. It is lined by an impervious layer of transitional epithelium which becomes thinner and flatter to accommodate the distension by the urine.

Microanatomy

Mucosa consists of **transitional epithelium**, 4–5 layers thick and thrown **into longitudinal folds to form a star shaped lumen with no glands opening into it**.

Lamina propria is wide consisting of fibroelastic tissue having diffuse lymphatic tissue.

Muscularis mucosae is absent.

Submucosa is not distinguishable.

Muscularis externa: The smooth muscle coat is thicker than mucosa is arranged in inner longitudinal, middle circular and outer longitudinal in the lower part. The reflux of the urine from the urinary bladder into the ureters is prevented by the oblique path followed by the terminal part of the ureter through the bladder wall and also by the contraction of smooth muscles.

Adventitia consists of loose collagenous fibers containing blood vessels and nerves. Since ureter is retroperitoneal so serosa i.e. mesothelial cells may be found over a portion of the periphery of the wall.

Keys for identification: Ureter

a. Mucosa thrown into longitudinal folds. Lumen is star shaped.
b. Lining epithelium is transitional.
c. Smooth muscle coat consists of 2–3 layers.

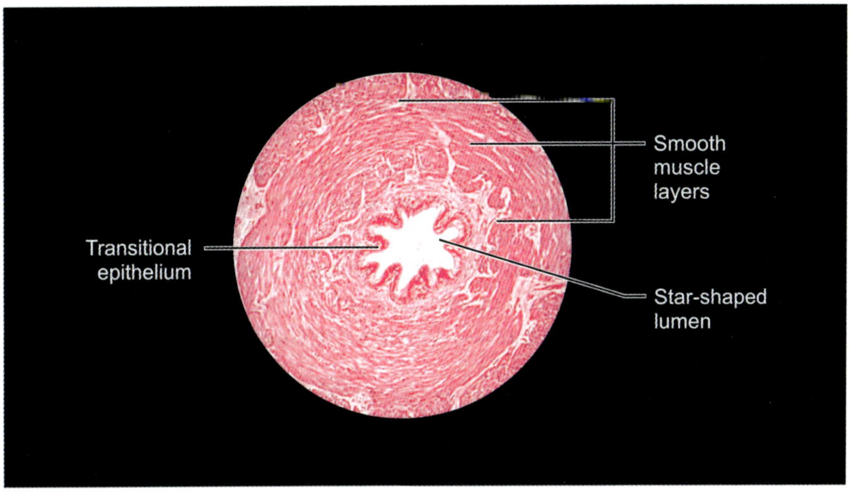

Fig. 3.33 Ureter

Blank space for sketch work by students

URINARY BLADDER (FIG. 3.34)

It receives the urine from the ureters and stores the urine until it is expelled out by neural stimulation through the urethra.

Microanatomy

The wall of the urinary bladder consists of:

- **Mucosa** is lined by transitional epithelium thrown into many folds in the relaxed state. The epithelium rests on a thin basement membrane.
- **Lamina propria** lies deep to the epithelium and contains capillaries, nuclei of fibroblasts, collagen and elastic fibers.
- **Muscularis externa** is thickest and the smooth muscle fibers are arranged as inner longitudinal middle circular and outer longitudinal but not seen as the description but arranged in all directions to exert equal pressure to expel the urine. Just above the junction of the bladder with the urethra the circular muscle coat is thickened to form the sphincter urethrae.
- **The serosa** or the **adventitia** is the outermost coat formed by mesothelial lining with the underlying connective tissue in case of serosa and loose connective tissue only in adventitia.

Keys for identification: Urinary bladder

a. Mucosa lined by transitional epithelium with no glands.
b. In the relaxed state mucosa is thrown into folds.
c. Smooth muscle fibers arranged in different planes.

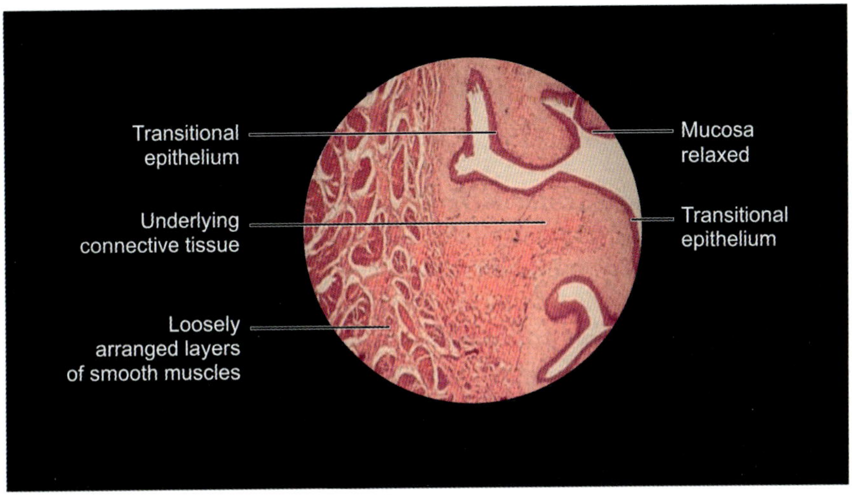

Fig. 3.34 Urinary bladder

Blank space for sketch work by students

URETHRA (FIG. 3.35)

The urethra is the passageway for urine and semen (sperm and associated secretions). Three regions of the urethra are distinguished:

- The **prostatic urethra** passes through the prostate gland.
- The **membranous urethra** passes through the urogenital diaphragm (muscles associated with the pelvic region).
- **The spongy (penile) urethra** passes through the penis.
  The urethra ends at the external urethral orifice.

Microanatomy

Mucosa is composed of:

- **Epithelium** is proximally lined by a **transitional epithelium** in males and females. In males, it is replaced by a pseudostratified or stratified columnar epithelium below the openings of the ejaculatory ducts into the urethra. The distal parts of the female urethra and the distal end of the male urethra are lined by a stratified squamous epithelium. Due to deep outpocketings of mucosa the outline of the **lumen is irregular**.
- **The lamina propria** contains loose connective tissue.
  Muscularis mucosae is absent.

Submucosa contains the erectile tissue which appear as broad **vascular lacunae** of corpus spongiosum around the lumen.

Muscularis externa: Smooth muscle cells are mainly oriented into inner longitudinal and outer circular layers. They are surrounded, in the middle part of the urethra (below the prostate in males), by striated muscle fibers of the sphincter urethrae and in females smooth muscle fibers are supplemented by striated muscle fibers.

Keys for identification: Urethra

a. Mucosa is lined by transitional or pseudostratified columnar or stratified columnar or stratified squamous epithelium.
b. Lumen is irregular.
c. Irregular venous spaces surround the lumen.

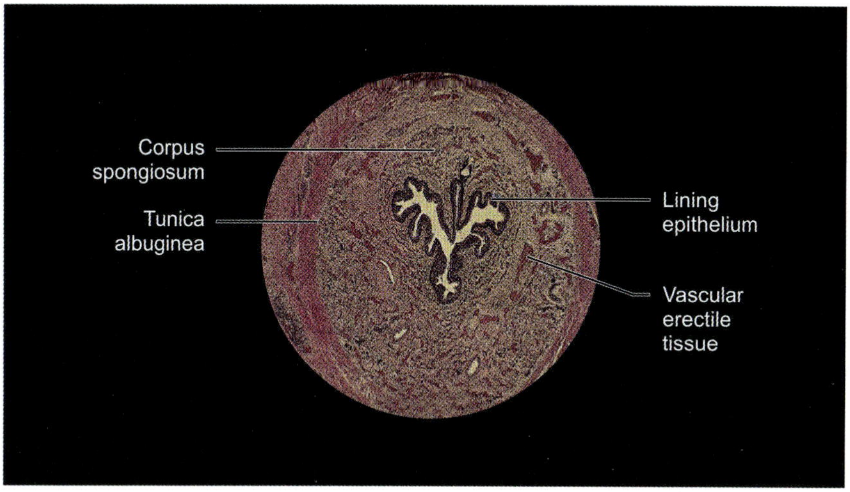

Fig. 3.35 Urethra

Blank space for sketch work by students

MALE REPRODUCTIVE SYSTEM

The **male reproductive system** consists of four main components.

1. The male sex organs are the testes:
   - Produce the male gametes.
   - Secrete testosterone.
2. **Genital ducts** include epididymis, vas deferens and ejaculatory duct. They collect, store and conduct spermatozoa from testes.
3. **Accessory glands** include seminal vesicles, prostate and bulbourethral glands which secrete seminal fluid.
4. **Organ of copulation**—Penis.

THE TESTIS (FIG. 3.36)

It consists of the following structures:

- The **tunica vaginalis** is a double-layered outer serous membrane surrounding each testis.
- The **tunica albuginea** lies inside the tunica vaginalis and protrudes inward, dividing each testis into compartments called lobules.
- Innermost is the **tunica vasculosa**.
- It is divided into about 250 pyramidal compartments called the lobules.
- Each lobule contains 1 to 4 tightly coiled tubules, the **seminiferous tubules**. The seminiferous tubules are the sites of sperm production (spermatogenesis) and lined with spermatogenic cells, which form sperm, and sustentacular cells (Sertoli cells), which support the developing sperm. The coiled seminiferous tubules inside each lobule unite to form a straight tube.
- The **rete testis** is a network of tubes formed by the merging of the straight tubules from each lobule.
- The **efferent ducts** transport sperms out of the testis (from the rete testis) to the epididymis.

Microanatomy

The parenchyma consists of the convoluted **seminiferous tubules**. These tubules are enclosed by a thick basal lamina and surrounded by 3–4 layers of smooth muscle cells. The tubules are lined with **seminiferous epithelium**, which consist of **spermatogenic cells** and **Sertoli cells**.

Spermatogenic Cells

The primordial germ cells are the first cells of spermatogenesis. They orginate in the endodermal walls of the yolk sac and migrate to the genital ridge, where they differentiate into spermatogonia. They remain dormant until puberty and in contact with the basal lamina of the tubule. Two types of cells are seen spermatogenic cells and nonspermatogenic cells called Sertoli cells in the seminiferous epithelium.

Type A spermatogonia have a rounded nucleus with very fine chromatin grains and one or two nucleoli. They are **stem cells** and maintain the germ cell pool, i.e. they are capable of continuous division, remain undifferentiated and never mature into specialized cells.

Type A divides to form new generations of both type A and type B spermatogonia.

Type B spermatogonia have rounded nuclei with chromatin granules of variable size attached to the nuclear membrane, and one nucleolus. Type B spermatogonia may divide repeatedly but do not function as stem cells and their division results in the formation of **primary spermatocytes**.

Primary spermatocytes migrate and lie in the adluminal compartment before starting the first meiotic division. They appear larger than spermatogonia. They immediately enter the prophase of the first meiotic division, which is extremely prolonged (about 22 days). A large number of primary spermatocytes are always visible in sections of seminiferous tubules. The completion of the first meiotic division results in the formation of **secondary spermatocytes**, which are smaller than primary spermatocytes.

Secondary spermatocytes rapidly enter and complete the second meiotic division and are therefore seldom seen in histological preparations. Their division results in the formation of **spermatids**, which lie towards the lumen of the seminiferous epithelium.

Spermatids are small (about 10 mm in diameter) with a very light (often eccentric) nucleus. The chromatin condenses during the maturation of the spermatids into spermatozoa, and the nucleus becomes smaller and stains darker.

The terminal phase of spermatogenesis is called spermiogenesis and consists of the differentiation of the newly formed spermatids into spermatozoa which are about 60 mm long and actively motile. It is divided into the following parts:

- The head of the sperm contains the haploid nucleus with 23 chromosomes. At the tip of the head is the acrosome, containing lysozymes that are used to penetrate the egg.
- The head is separated from the middle piece by a narrow **neck**.
- The middle piece is the first part of the tail. Mitochondria spiral around the middle piece and produce energy (ATP) used to generate the whip like movements of the tail that propel the sperm.
- The tail is a flagellum consisting of the typical 9 + 2 microtubule array.

Sertoli cells are less numerous than spermatogenic cells and are evenly distributed between them. Their shape is highly irregular generally columnar extending from the basement membrane to the luminal surface of the seminiferous epithelium. Processes of the Sertoli cells extend in between the spermatogenic cells (cell limits are therefore not clearly visible in the LM). The nucleus of Sertoli cells is ovoid or angular, large and lightly stained and often contains a large nucleolus. The long axis of the nucleus is oriented perpendicular to wall of the tubule.

Lateral processes of Sertoli cells are interconnected by tight junctions, which form the **blood-testis barrier** and divide the tubule into the basal and the adluminal compartment. Spermatogonia and primary spermatocytes are located in the basal compartment, other cellular stages of spermatogenesis are located in the adluminal compartment. Tight junctions may temporarily open to permit the passage of primary spermatocytes from the basal into the adluminal compartment. Sertoli cells provide mechanical and nutritive support for the spermatogenic cells. Sertoli cells also secrete two hormones-inhibin and activin which provide positive and negative feedback of follicle stimulating hormone (FSH) secretion from the pituitary. Spermatogenesis is regulated by FSH, which in males stimulates spermatogenic epithelium, and luteinizing-hormone (LH), which in males stimulates testosterone production by Leydig cells in the interstitial tissue. These cells also produce androgen binding protein.

Interstitial tissue contains fibroblasts, nerves, blood and lymph vessels and endocrine component of testis is formed by Leydig cells (15–20 mm), located in the interstitial tissue between the convoluted seminiferous tubules. They synthesize and secrete testosterone. Leydig cells occur in clusters, which are variable in size and richly supplied by capillaries. The cytoplasm is strongly acidophilic and finely granular. The nucleus is large, round and often located eccentric in the cell and contains fat droplets in the cytoplasm. It may contain rod shaped "crystals of Reinke".

Keys for identification: Testis

a. A large number of seminiferous tubules are seen.
b. Spermatogenic cells and Sertoli cells are seen.
c. Presence of Leydig cells.

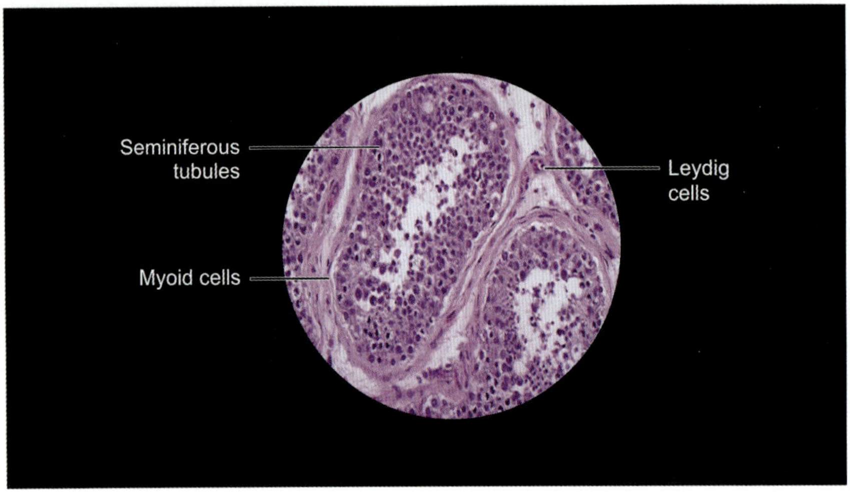

Fig. 3.36 Testis

Blank space for sketch work by students

EPIDIDYMIS (FIG. 3.37)

- The epididymis is a comma-shaped organ that lies adjacent to each testis and has three parts head, body and tail.
- The epididymis consists of a highly convoluted tube where maturation of sperms is completed and the sperms stored until ejaculation.
- During ejaculation smooth muscles encircling the epididymis contract, forcing mature sperms into the ductus deferens.
- The major function of the epididymis is accumulation, storage and maturation of sperms.

Microanatomy

Mucosa

- A number of tubules of varying size and shape surrounded by connective tissue are seen.
  The tubules are lined by pseudostratified columnar epithelium with stereocilia.
  Two types of cells are seen:
  1. Columnar with elongated nuclei located at a distance from the base of the cells and having nonmotile stereocilia on the free surface. These cells are secretory in nature and nourish the sperms present in the lumen. These stereocilia absorb testicular fluid, remove the degenerated sperms and secrete a glycoprotein which inhibits capacitation of sperms in the male reproductive tract.
  2. Basal cells with round nucleus close to the basement membrane.
- Because of the unusual height of the columnar cells and tortuosity of ducts the lumen is uneven and at some places even islands of epithelium are seen in the lumen.
- Sperms may be seen in the lumen.
- A thin layer of smooth muscles surrounds the tubules in a circular manner which helps to move the sperm along the ducts. Movement of the sperm is also brought about by the vacuum created by the absorption of fluid and cellular debris.

Keys for identification: Epididymis

a. Tubules lined by pseudostratified columnar epithelium with stereocilia seen.
b. In the lumen sperms are seen.
c. Smooth muscle fibers surround the tubules.

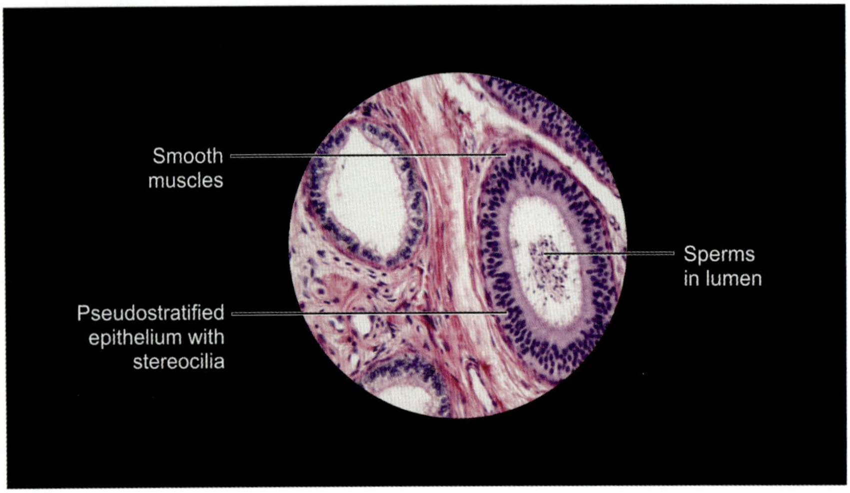

Fig. 3.37 Epididymis

Blank space for sketch work by students

VAS DEFERENS (FIG. 3.38)

Vas deferens is a long, narrow tube that carries sperm from the epididymis to the seminal vesicles during ejaculation.

Microanatomy

- It is the tube through which sperms travel when they leave the epididymis and together with the duct of the seminal vesicle forms the ejaculatory duct. Sperms are stored in the ductus deferens until peristaltic contractions of the smooth muscles surrounding the ductus deferens force sperms forward during ejaculation.
- There is no **submucosa**.
- **Muscularis** is composed of smooth muscles which are arranged as a thick outer longitudinal layer, a thick circular layer and a thin inner longitudinal layer.
- **Adventitia** is made up of loose connective tissue containing blood vessels and nerves.

Keys for identification: Vas deferens

a. Mucosa lined by pseudostratified columnar epithelium with stereocilia.
b. Thick muscle coat.
c. Stellate lumen.

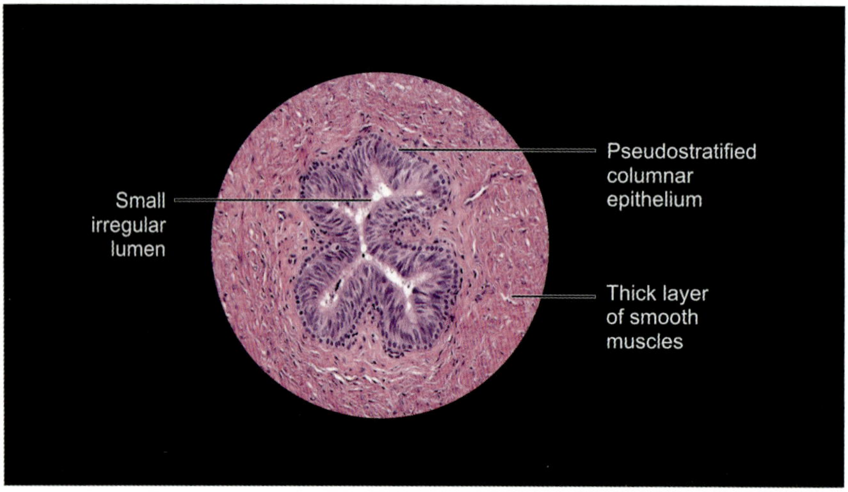

Fig. 3.38 Vas deferens

Blank space for sketch work by students

SEMINAL VESICLES (FIG. 3.38A)

It is a complex glandular diverticulum of ductus deferens. It secretes up to 85% of seminal fluid and the rest is being secreted by the prostate. It is a tightly coiled tube so the lumen is highly irregular and many recesses may be seen giving a honeycomb appearance.

The seminal vesicles secrete into the vas deferens an alkaline fluid (which neutralizes the acid in the vagina), fructose (which provides energy for the sperm), and prostaglandins (which increase sperm viability and stimulate female uterine contractions that help sperm move into the uterus).

Microanatomy

- **Mucosa** is thrown into folds which branch and anastomose giving a **honeycomb appearance**.
- The epithelial lining is **pseudostratified** tall columnar or **simple columnar to cuboidal** depending on the secretory activity.
- Lamina propria contains many elastic fibers thrown into complex mucosal folds of mucous membrane which branch and anastomose giving the lumen a honeycomb appearance.
- The cells are secretory in type with lipid droplets giving it a foamy appearance.
- A few sperms may be seen which might have entered due to reflux from the ampulla. The connective tissue contains blood vessels and nerves.

Keys for identification: Seminal vesicles

a. Mucosa is highly branched having anastomosing folds.
b. No sperms in the lumen.
c. Well-developed muscle layer is seen.

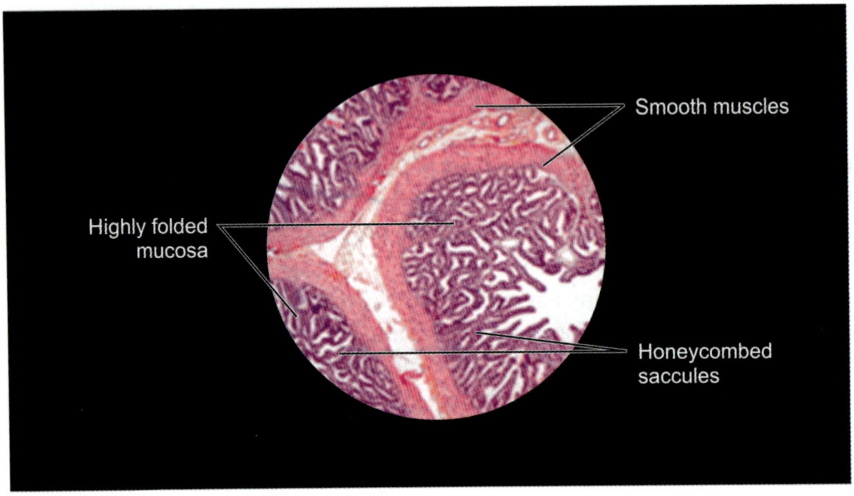

Fig. 3.38A Seminal vesicles

Blank space for sketch work by students

PROSTATE GLAND (FIG. 3.39)

It is the largest accessory sex gland. It is a compound tubuloalveolar type of gland which is embedded in a fibromuscular stoma. It is surrounded by a capsule composed of elastic fibers and some smooth muscle fibers. This gland is also responsible for making the semen milky by mixing calcium to the fluid coming from seminal vesicle. Prostatic fluid is thin watery and slightly acidic containing acid phosphatase, amylase and citric acid which provide nutrition to sperms and neutralizes the acidity of vagina. Various substances in the fluid increase sperm mobility and viability.

Microanatomy

- The acini are irregular in shape with folded epithelium which projects into the lumen along with some connective tissue forming folds to allow for expansion of the glands by secretions.
- Epithelial lining is made up of double layer of cells. The cells towards the lumen are tall columnar secretory cells with basal nuclei.
- Between the secretory cells and the basement membrane lies a layer of basal cells which act as reserve cells to replace the secretory cells.
- The lumen of the acini are sometimes filled with small colloid masses known as corpora amylacea or amyloid bodies, which are the aggregations of dead epithelial cells and precipitated secretory products.
- They appear as uniform or lamellated structures consisting of condensed glycoprotein which is often calcified.
- The stroma consists of dense collagen fibers and smooth muscle fibers which produce powerful contractions during ejaculation.

Keys for identification: Prostate gland

a. Irregular acini with epithelium folded inwards seen.
b. The stroma is fibromuscular.
c. The acini are filled with corpora amylacea.

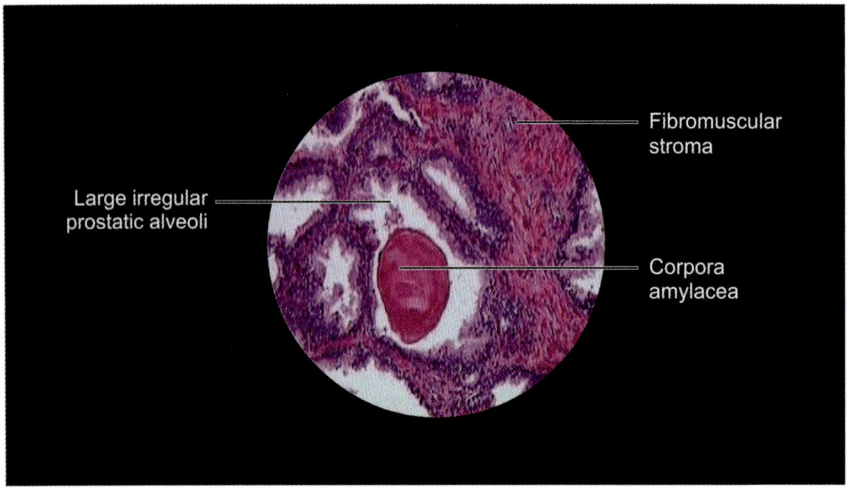

Fig. 3.39 Prostate gland

Blank space for sketch work by students

PENIS (FIG. 3.40)

The penis is the male copulatory organ. It acts as a passage for both urine and sperms. Dermis is composed of smooth muscle fibers and dilated venous spaces. Internally penis consists of three cylindrical masses of erectile tissue, each of which is surrounded by a thin layer of fibrous tissue, the **tunica albuginea**. Two **corpora cavernosa** fill most of the volume of the penis. Single corpus spongiosum encloses the urethra.

Microanatomy

- The penis is covered by a **thin skin** devoid of hair follicles.
- Deep to this is loose connective tissue devoid of fat called **Buck's fascia** which allows free movement of skin and contains elastic fibers, smooth muscle fibers and dorsal vein, dorsal artery and nerve.
- The penis consists of three cylindrical masses of erectile tissue.
- They include paired **corpora cavernosa** on the dorsal aspect and the midline **corpus spongiosum** which surrounds and supports the penile urethra ventrally.
- **Tunica albuginea** surrounds each corpora cavernosa which comprises of trabeculae of connective tissue and smooth muscle fibers enclosing spaces or caverns which are lined by endothelial cells. These vascular sinuses are supplied by thick walled helicine arteries (as they follow a spiral course) and drained by venules. In the corpus spongiosum, trabeculae are finer and branches of helicine arteries are narrow.

Mature/Graafian follicle: The granulosa cells now consist of many layers of cuboidal follicular epithelial cells located at the periphery of the large, well formed follicular antrum. The oocyte has attained its full size, is located eccentrically within the follicle in a small hillock, the **cumulus oophorus** which protrudes into the antrum. The zona pellucida is surrounded by a continuous layer of follicular cells, the **corona radiata**. The size of oocyte is small so it is not seen in every section of the follicle.

The theca interna is separated from the granulosa cells by a distinct basement membrane. Theca externa cells are densely packed, spindle-shaped cells that blend with the theca interna cells having a **rich capillary vascular supply** and with the surrounding stroma.

Atretic follicles: Only one follicle usually ovulates at a time, other follicles which have been stimulated to develop must degenerate, or undergo atresia. Atresia is not limited to mature follicles, but may begin at any stage in follicular development. Early atretic changes include clumping of the nuclear chromatin (pyknosis) and shrinkage and lysis of the cytoplasm of the oocyte, granulosa or follicular cells. The basement membrane that separates the granulosa cells from the theca interna may also thicken considerably to form the "**glassy membrane**". Macrophages may eventually invade the center of the larger atretic follicles that are finally replaced by loose connective tissue.

Corpus luteum: It is the remains of the follicle following ovulation.

- After ovulation, the follicle collapses and becomes highly infolded and invaded by vessels, forming the corpus luteum (yellow body).
- It appears pale and highly folded. If the egg is fertilized and implanted, the corpus luteum enlarges to become the **corpus luteum of pregnancy**.
- The inner **granulosa lutein** cells are formed from the remaining granulosa cells and the outer theca **lutein cells** which come from the remaining **theca interna** cells. Both cell types are polyhedral and filled with lipid droplets and have centrally located nuclei.
- The **theca lutein** cells are small more darkly stained and have fewer lipid filled cells than the granulosa lutein cells. They are found most prominently in the infoldings right up against the granulosa lutein layer.
- Granulosa lutein cells contain a pigment lipochrome, which produce the yellowish color of the corpus luteum. A central blood clot may be present in recently ovulated follicles.
- It remains functional if fertilization takes place, producing estrogen, progesterone, and inhibin until it finally degenerates and the function is taken over by the placenta.

Corpus albicans: If the oocyte is not fertilized, the corpus luteum degenerates, and is gradually infiltrated with collagen and a few fibroblasts, forming the **corpus albicans** (white body). The corpus albicans is also formed during the later half of pregnancy when the placenta takes over steroid secretion from the corpus luteum.

Keys for identification: Ovary—(1)

a. Mucosa lined by cuboidal epithelium.
b. Deep to this is tunica albuginea.
c. Cortex containing various stages of developing follicles.
d. Medulla contains connective tissue and blood vessels.

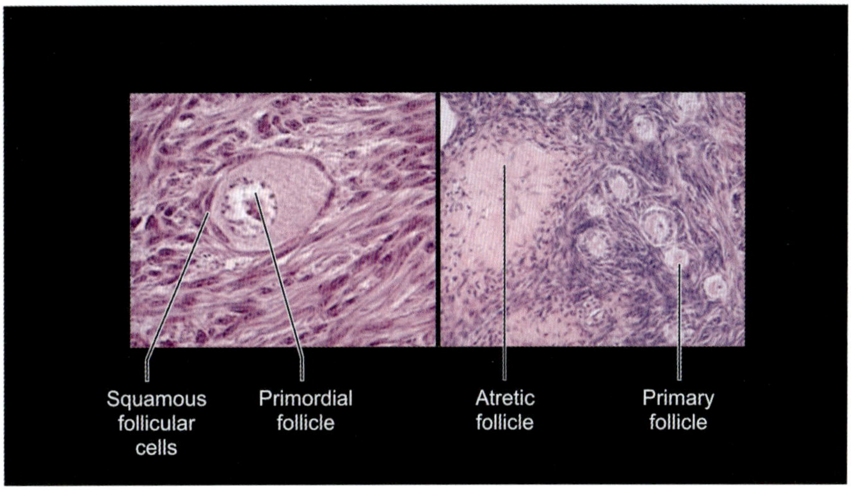

Fig. 3.41 Ovary—(1)

Blank space for sketch work by students

Keys for identification: Ovary—(2)

a. Germinal epithelium overlies tunica albuginea.
b. Various types of maturing follicles seen.
c. Outer cortex and inner medulla without distinct boundaries seen.

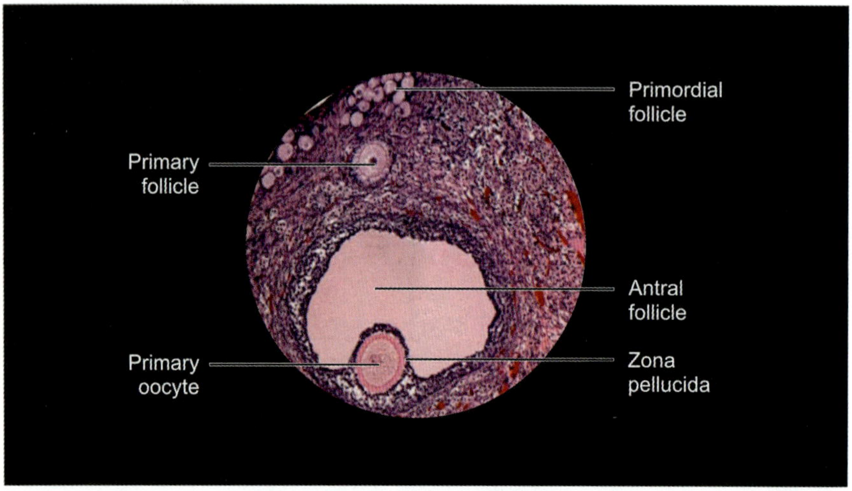

Fig. 3.42 Ovary—(2)

Blank space for sketch work by students

THE UTERINE TUBES (OVIDUCTS) (FIG. 3.43)

They transport the ovum (secondary oocytes) away from the ovary towards the uterus within three days during which fertilization of ovum and segmentation of zygote occurs. The following four regions are seen:

1. The **infundibulum** is a funnel-shaped region of the uterine tube that bears finger like projections called fimbriae. Pulsating cilia on the fimbriae draw the secondary oocyte into the uterine tube.
2. The **ampulla** is the widest and longest region of the uterine tube which has the thickest muscle coat.
3. The **isthmus** is a narrow region of the uterine tube which has the thickest muscle coat.
4. The **intramural** part that passes through the thick uterine wall.

Microanatomy

The wall of the uterine tube consists of the following three layers:

1. **The serosa** is the outermost layer, highly vascular and lined by mesothelial cells.
2. The middle **muscularis externa** consists of two layers of smooth muscles inner circular and outer longitudinal that generate peristaltic contractions which help propel the oocyte forward towards the uterus from the peritoneal cavity.
3. The inner **mucosa** is thrown into a labyrinth of branching folds which occupy the entire lumen without any anastomosis.

The epithelial lining consists of three types of cells.

1. Ciliated cells that move like a wave towards the uterus. Ciliated cells are shorter than secretory cells making the surface lining irregular.
2. Nonciliated secretory cells called peg cells produce a secretion that provides nutrition and protection to the ovum.
3. **Intercalated** cells are the variant of secretory cells.

Keys for identification: Uterine tube

a. Mucosa thrown into labyrinth of branching folds.
b. Muscular layer consists of inner circular and outer longitudinal layers.
c. Serosa is the outermost layer.

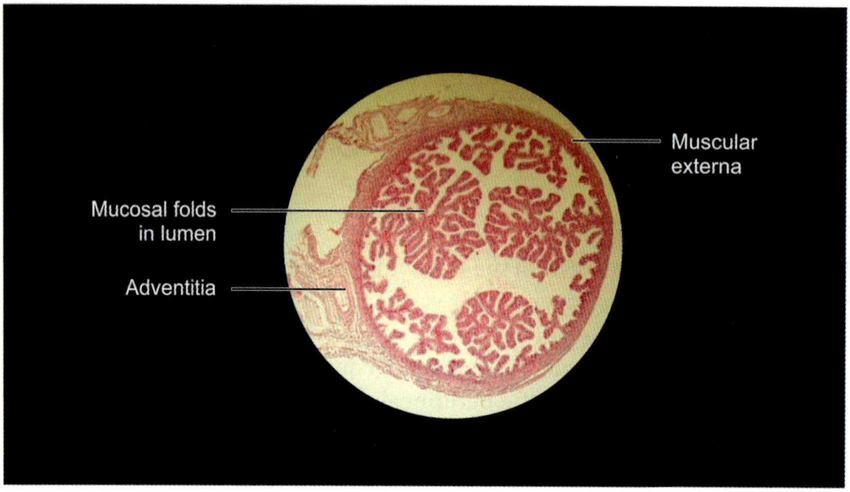

Fig. 3.43 Uterine tube

Blank space for sketch work by students

THE UTERUS (FIGS 3.44 TO 3.46)

It is a pear-shaped, hollow organ partially covered by peritoneum.

Microanatomy

- **Outer serosal or adventitial covering**—serosa is a thin fibrous tissue layer covered by mesothelial cells.
- **Adventitia** consists of an outer layer of loose connective tissue rich in blood vessels, lymph vessels and adipose tissue.

Thick muscular layer (Myometrium)

The myometrium of the uterus is composed of interwoven bundles of smooth muscles running roughly parallel to the long axis of the body of the uterus and supported by dense connective tissue. During pregnancy, the muscle fibers elongate, proliferate and produce collagen in response to hormonal stimulation.

Mucosa (Endometrium)

- The mucosa is lined by **simple columnar ciliated epithelium**.
- The underlying stroma contains **simple tubular glands**.
- The **stratum functionale** or functional layer is the thicker, outer layer that is sloughed off with menstruation.
- The underlying basal layer is retained throughout the menstrual cycle and serves as the regenerative source of the stratum functionale.
- The endometrium undergoes cyclical changes during the proliferative and secretory phases of the menstrual cycle.
  - *Proliferative phase (4–14 days):* The glands have proliferated and cover the surface.

    The **spiral arteries** are elongated, convoluted and extend from the basal layer into the functional layer.
  - *Secretory phase (days 15-28):* The glands of the endometrium appear convoluted.

    Toward the end of this phase, apical tissues become ischemic and glands take on a **characteristic "saw tooth" appearance**.

    The endometrium reaches its maximal thickness during this period, and **spiral arteries** continue to grow and extend into the superficial regions of the functional layer.

    There is also considerable leukocyte infiltration in the stroma.
  - *Menstrual phase (days 1-4),* much of the stratum functionale is sloughed off, the debris includes numerous blood cells (RBCs and leukocytes), whereas the **stratum basale** remains intact.

Keys for identification: Uterus (Menstrual phase)

a. Mucosa lined by simple columnar ciliated epithelium.
b. Simple tubular glands seen in lamina propria.
c. Myometrium is thick with presence of arterioles.

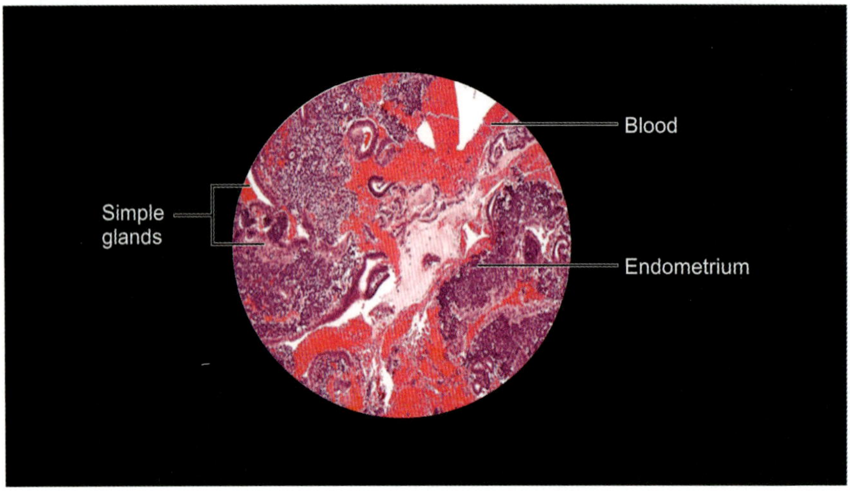

Fig. 3.44 Uterus (Menstrual phase)

Blank space for sketch work by students

Keys for identification: Uterus (Proliferative phase)

a. Very thick muscle layer with numerous blood vessels.
b. Mucous membrane (endometrium) lined by simple columnar epithelium.
c. Lamina propria containing simple tubular uterine glands. 'Straight glands'

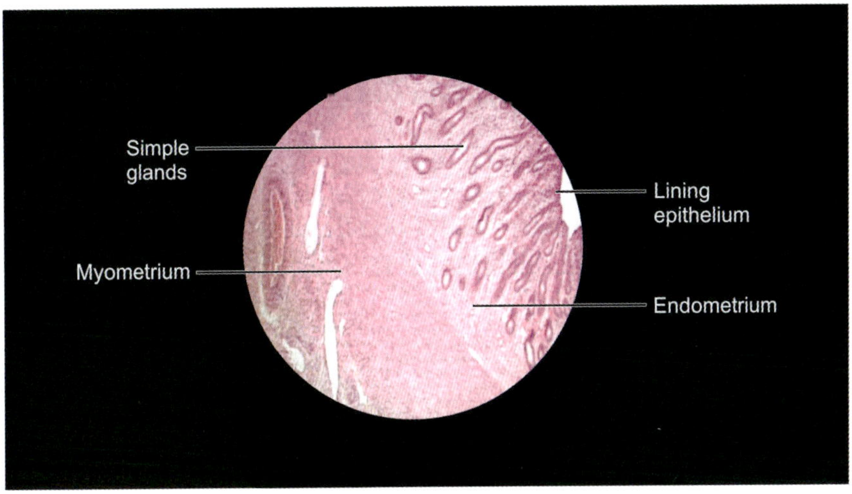

Fig. 3.45 Uterus (Proliferative phase)

Blank space for sketch work by students

Keys for identification: Vagina

a. Lined by stratified squamous nonkeratinized epithelium.
b. No glands.
c. Numerous elastic fibers present in adventitia.

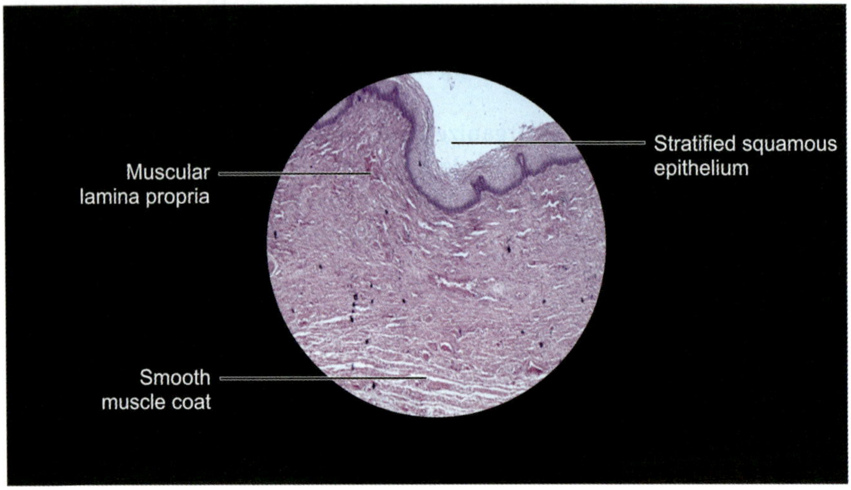

Fig. 3.47 Vagina

Blank space for sketch work by students

PLACENTA (FIG. 3.48)

It is specialized extra embryonic tissue where fetal blood vessels come in contact with maternal blood only separated by placental membrane for the purpose of nutrition, respiration, excretion and other metabolic functions.

Microanatomy

With the implantation of a zygote into the uterus, a number of changes take place in the endometrium.

Cells from the embryonic trophoblast invade the uterine mucosa, which is now termed the **decidua**. The trophoblast rapidly invades the decidua forming primary villus that contains only trophoblast (outer **syncytiotrophoblast** and inner cytotrophoblast) cells.

Mesenchyme forms the core of the secondary villi. Fetal blood vessels filled with fetal RBCs which have nuclei are seen in the tertiary villi. Maternal blood is present in the intervillous space. During the second half of pregnancy the cytotrophoblast cells disappear and the capillary basal lamina fuses with that of the syncytiotrophoblast to improve exchange.

Mesenchymal tissue is covered by a trophectoderm shell of inner cytotrophoblast and outer syncytiotrophoblast cells. The syncytiotrophoblast cells are more eosinophilic and have smaller nuclei. These cells result from the fusion of many cells and thus have many nuclei per cell and no clear lateral boundaries. In contrast, cytotrophoblast cells have a single, large nucleus and basophilic cytoplasm. On the outer surface of the villi multinucleate syncytiotrophoblast cells are located. The nuclei of the syncytiotrophoblast cells often form aggregates of "**syncytial knots**". Syncytiotrophoblast cells are bathed in maternal blood which have apical surfaces specialized for absorption (microvilli), pinocytosis, and exocytosis and an appearance typical of secretory cells. Numerous macrophage-like (Hofbauer) cells can be found within the connective tissue of the placental villi. These cells are characteristically large, with elliptical, eccentric nuclei and extensively vacuolated cytoplasm.

Large quantities of an amorphous eosinophilic substance, **fibrinoid** may also be deposited in the intervillus space in the older placenta. This material clings to the villus surface and may bind several villi together.

Keys for identification: Placenta

a. The villi are lined by an epithelium having an inner layer of cytotrophoblast and outer layer of syncytiotrophoblast.
b. These villi contain fetal capillaries with nucleated RBCs and fetal connective tissue in the core of the villus.
c. Maternal blood is present in the intervillous space.

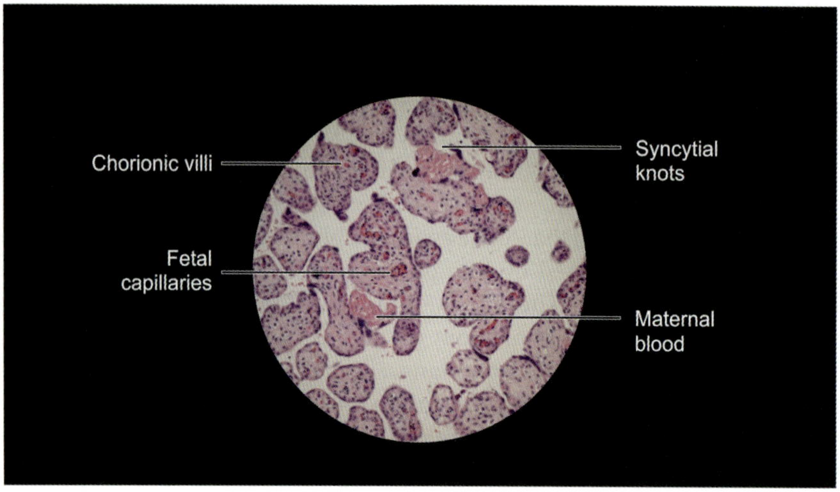

Fig. 3.48 Placenta

Blank space for sketch work by students

UMBILICAL CORD (FIG. 3.49)

It is a 50 cm long tubular structure connecting the fetus with the placenta.

Microanatomy

- Consists of an outer covering of flattened amniotic **epithelial** cells.
- This surrounds the central mass of viscid mucoid connective tissue known as **Wharton's jelly**.
- Fibroblasts are seen separated by fine collagen fibers and ground substance.
- Traversing in the cord are **two umbilical arteries and single left umbilical vein**.
- The arteries are identified by small, regular and round lumen, thick walled muscle coat with prominent and folded internal elastic lamina.
- Vein shows a thin folded, collapsed irregular lumen and thick adventitia.

Keys for identification: Umbilical cord

a. Outer covering of flattened amniotic epithelial cells.
b. Core of mesoderm undergoes mucoid degeneration forming Wharton's jelly.
c. Traversing the cord are two umbilical arteries and a single left umbilical vein.

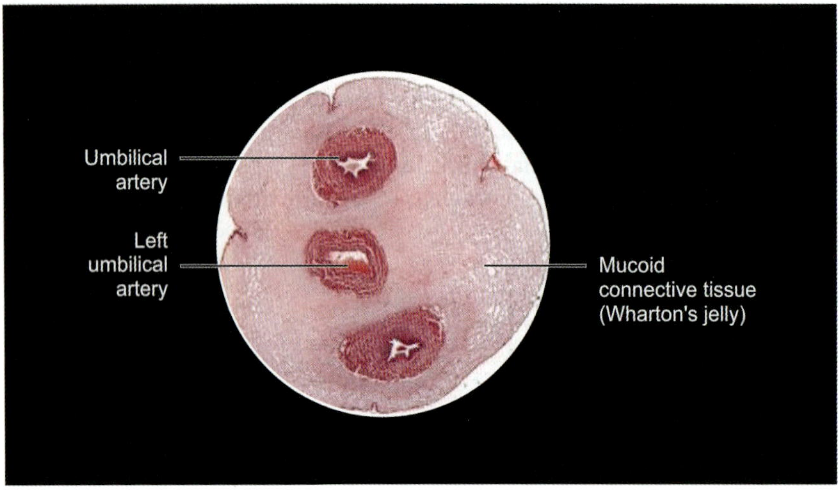

Fig. 3.49 Umbilical cord

Blank space for sketch work by students

MAMMARY GLANDS (FIGS 3.50 AND 3.51)

The mammary glands are compound tubuloalveolar type of glands specialized for milk production. The milk-producing secretory cells called alveoli join together with ducts, in grapelike fashion, to form lobules. Numerous lobules join to form a lobe (total 15–20 lobes). These lobes are separated by a interlobular dense fibrofatty stroma (differentiated from prostate gland where the stroma is fibromuscular). The lobes drain into lactiferous ducts.

Microanatomy

In nonlactating breast dense irregular interlobular connective tissue is seen between lobules that consist of only a few clusters of small ducts lined with cuboidal or low columnar cells surrounded by a mass of less dense intralobular connective tissue. Many ducts appear to be composed of two layers of cuboidal epithelium (stratified). The inner layer is the actual ductal epithelial cells whereas the outer layer of cells is a layer of myoepithelial cells. The glandular tissue is scanty, alveoli are not developed and represented by solid cords of epithelial cells. Lobule is formed by extensive division of duct system. Interlobular connective tissue is thick and fibrofatty in nature. There is increased intralobular connective tissue containing fibroblasts.

In the lactating breast the amount of the glandular tissue has increased, while the interlobular connective tissue is reduced to a thin septum. A large number of distended alveoli which are irregular in shape filled with milk secretion are seen. This increase involves the numbers of both the epithelial cells and myoepithelial cells. Active alveoli are lined by low epithelium and filled with eosinophilic material whereas inactive alveoli have empty lumen and tall epithelium. The intralobular ducts lined by cuboidal epithelium can be differentiated from the alveoli by being more regular. The lactiferous ducts are lined by stratified columnar or cuboidal epithelium.

The intralobular ducts have proliferated to form additional secretory regions. Some alveolar cells accumulate glycogen and lipid in the apical cytoplasm and they appear to have large, clear areas because fat is removed during the routine tissue processing. The epithelial lining is again two layered, the bottom layer being formed by myoepithelial cells which contract to expel milk from the alveoli into the interlobular excretory duct lying in the interlobular connective tissue. The interlobular duct also contains the secretion so is difficult to differentiate from the alveoli, except that the lining epithelium is of stratified columnar cells.

Keys for identification: Lactating breast

a. Large number of distended alveoli filled with milk are seen.
b. Interlobular connective tissue is reduced to a thin septum.
c. Excretory ducts are seen in the interlobular connective tissue.

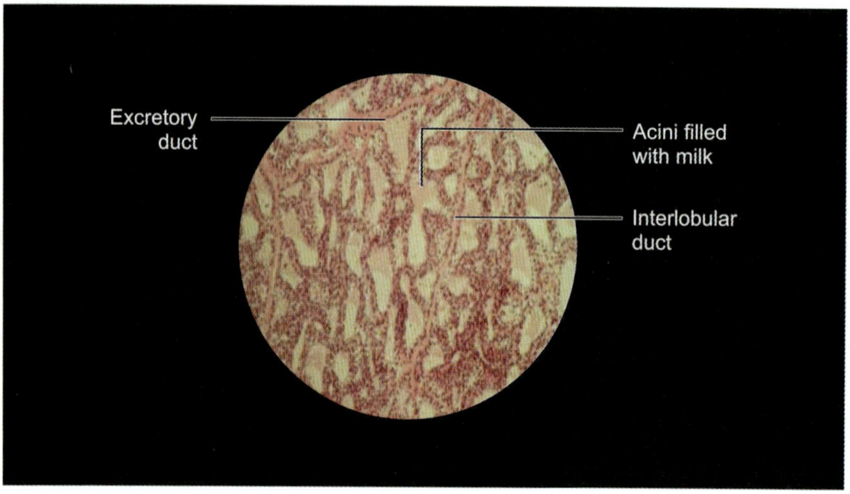

Fig. 3.50 Mammary gland (Lactating)

Blank space for sketch work by students

Keys for identification: Nonlactating breast

a. Few ducts lined by cuboidal or low columnar cells are seen.
b. Interlobular connective tissue is more dense and fibrofatty.
c. Absence of alveoli filled with milk.

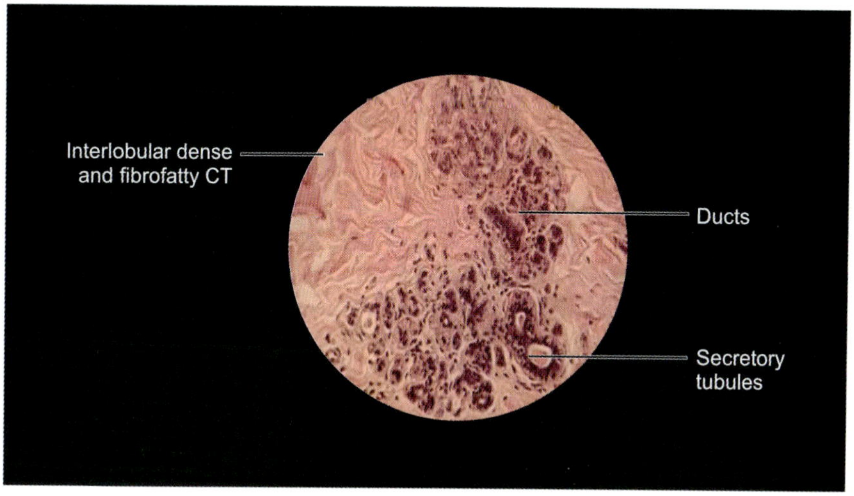

Fig. 3.51 Mammary gland (Nonlactating)

Blank space for sketch work by students

ENDOCRINE SYSTEM

THE ENDOCRINE GLANDS

These are the **ductless glands**. The epithelial cells are not arranged around ducts but in close association with blood capillaries so cell products (hormones) are rapidly absorbed by the circulatory system. The pancreas (islets of Langerhans), kidneys (J.G. cells and Lacis cells), testes (Leydig cells), ovaries (ovarian follicle and corpus luteum), placenta (chorion), brain, lungs and GIT (enteroendocrinal cells) are known to produce hormones but they have other functions also (endocrinal tissue is found in association with other organs). Some organs are totally endocrinal glands in function i.e. pituitary, thyroid, pineal, parathyroid and adrenal gland.

THYROID GLAND (FIG. 3.52)

It lies in the neck region, its function is to synthesize, store and release the thyroid hormones, thyroxine (T_4) and tri-iodothyronine (T_3) whenever required from the colloid and then stored in an inactive form. Thyroid hormones are necessary for the growth and metabolism of the body.

The thyroid gland is covered by two capsules, outer false fascial and inner true fibroelastic capsule which send septae inwards to divide the gland into lobules. These septa provide support to the fenestrated capillaries.

Microanatomy

Thyroid gland is composed of **parenchyma** in the form of follicles and **stroma** in the form of connective tissue interspersed with capillaries.

It is composed of many irregular and spherical functional units called **thyroid follicles** (both active and resting follicles are seen).

Each follicle is lined by **cuboidal epithelium** consisting of follicular or principal cells. The center of each follicle contains colloid secreted by the follicular cells. The colloid is composed of **thyroglobulin**. The quantity and consistency of the colloid and the shape of the cells in the epithelium depend on the functional activity of the gland. In the presence of low levels of thyroid stimulating hormone (TSH) the follicular cells are **squamous** and the colloid is dense and abundant (gland is hypoactive) and the size of the follicle is large. When stimulated by high levels of TSH the cells of the epithelium become more **columnar** and the amount of colloid is reduced (gland is hyperactive) stains less intensely and may appear vacuolated or "foamy" around the periphery and follicle is small in size. The secretory activity of follicular cells is controlled by TSH of adenohypophysis.

Between these follicles or lying between follicular cells and basement membrane are the **parafollicular cells** (derived from the neural crest) these cells are larger and less intensely stained than the follicular cells. They are called C cells or clear cells. They produce calcitonin in direct response to raised blood calcium levels and are not dependent on pituitary or parathyroid hormones. It lowers the raised blood calcium levels by suppressing bone resorption by osteoclasts.

Keys for identification: Thyroid gland

a. Thyroid follicles lined by cuboidal epithelium are seen.
b. Lumen filled with eosinophilic colloid material.
c. Parafollicular cells seen.

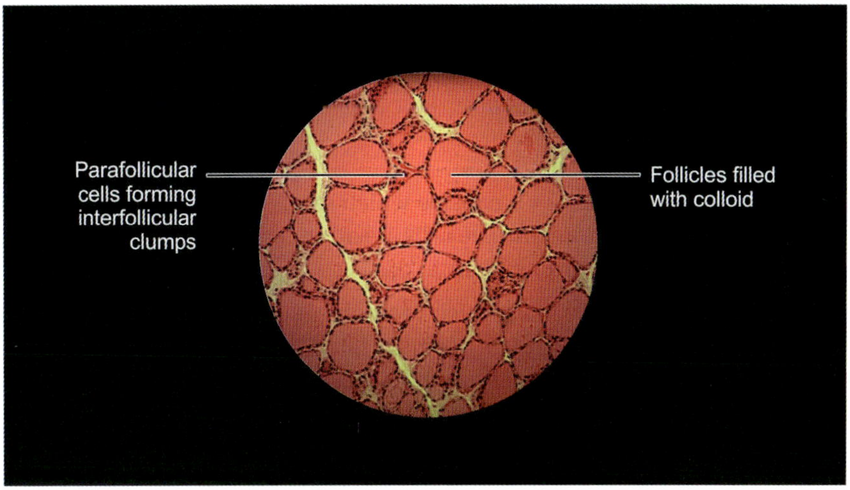

Fig. 3.52 Thyroid gland

Blank space for sketch work by students

THE PARATHYROID GLAND (FIG. 3.53)

Its function is to regulate calcium and phosphate levels. It secretes a hormone called parathormone. PTH increases the number and activity of the osteoclasts. This causes resorption of the calcified bone matrix and release of calcium and phosphate in the blood. PTH and calcitonin have opposite effects and they form a dual mechanism to regulate the blood calcium level. It also stimulates the kidneys to form calcitriol which is the active form of vitamin D. This increases the absorption of calcium from the gut. In the kidneys, it stimulates the absorption of calcium by the tubules. Urinary phosphate excretion is increased resulting into lower concentration of phosphate in the blood.

Microanatomy

Each parathyroid gland is covered by a capsule which sends septae that merge with reticular fibers which support the secretory cells. The cells are arranged in the form of thick anastomosing cords. There is no follicular arrangement.

Chief cells or principal cells (60–70%) which are polygonal in shape with rounded, central nucleus and pale staining eosinophilic cytoplasm filled with secretory granules containing parathyroid hormone (PTH) called parathormone. It regulates blood calcium level.

Oxyphil cells (30–40%) are much larger than principal cells characterized by acidophilic cytoplasm and dark prominent small and central nucleus. Some cells synthesize low levels of PTH in pathological conditions suggesting that they are the derivatives of chief cells.

Keys for identification: Parathyroid gland

a. Small chief cells seen.
b. Large oxyphil cells with eosinophilic cytoplasm present.
c. May be accompanied by thyroid tissue.

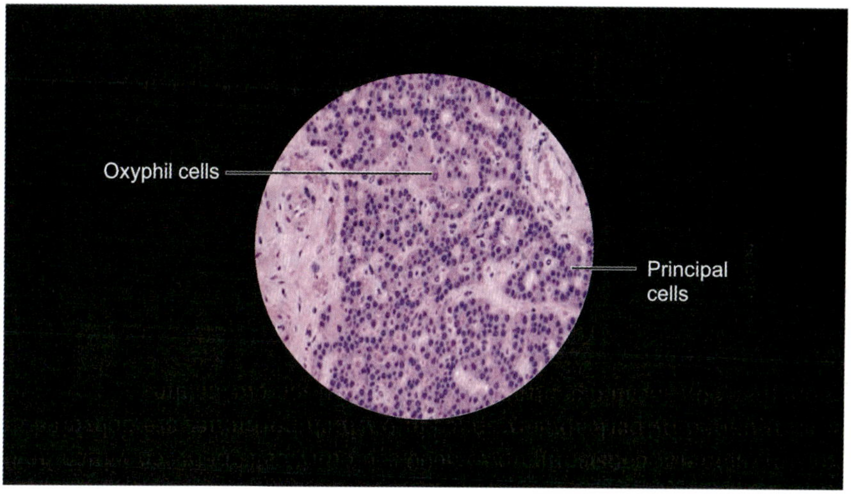

Fig. 3.53 Parathyroid gland

Blank space for sketch work by students

PITUITARY GLAND (FIG. 3.54)

It is known as the **master gland**. Some of the hormones secreted by it control the secretory activity of other endocrine glands. Its own activity is under the control of regulatory hormones produced by the hypothalamus. It is developed from two different types of epithelium, i.e. oral ectoderm which forms Rathke's pouch and neural ectoderm from the base of the diencephalon. Pituitary gland has two functional components.

Neurohypophysis: The posterior lobe consists of neurosecretory tissue. It includes:

- Median eminence.
- Infundibular stalk.
- Pars nervosa (infundibular process).

This region consists of unmyelinated nerve fibers (axons). Cell bodies are in the hypothalamus and these nerve fibers carry oxytocin and antidiuretic hormone to nerve ending and the hormones are stored in the expanded nerve terminal portion of nerve fibers. ADH antidiuretic hormone (vasopressin) is synthesized by neurons in the supraoptic nucleus of the hypothalamus. Oxytocin is synthesized by neurons in the paraventricular nucleus of the hypothalamus. The stored neurosecretory material appears as Herring bodies from where they are released into nearby capillaries upon neural stimulation from the hypothalamus.

Adenohypophysis: The anterior lobe includes:

- Pars distalis
- Pars intermedia
- Pars tuberalis.

Pars distalis: is organized as cords or clusters of cells supported by reticular connective tissue. Two types of cells can be observed:

1. **Chromophils** are 50% which stain red (acidophils), larger in size, lie at the periphery in close association with the sinusoids, others are stained blue (basophils) depending on the type of secretory material present, and
2. **Chromophobes** (50%) which do not take up the stain and thus appear unstained or clear. Chromophobes may be chromophils that have lost their secretory granules or chromophils that have not accumulated large numbers of secretory granules.

Acidophilic cells are:

- *Somatotrophs* secrete growth hormone which affects many cells.
- *Mammotrophs* secrete prolactin which controls milk production during lactation.

Basophilic cells are:

- *Corticotrophs* secrete ACTH which controls secretion of cortisol by cells in the adrenal cortex.
- *MSH* controls skin pigmentation.
- *Thyrotrophs* secrete TSH which controls secretion of thyroid gland (T_3 and T_4).
- *Gonadotrophs* secrete FSH which control development of follicles in females and spermiogenesis in males and LH (ICSH) regulates ovulation in the ovary and stimulation of Leydig cells to secrete testosterone in males.

Pars intermedia: The cells in the pars intermedia stain blue-purple and are basophilic with colloid filled spaces in between. In lower animals, it produces MSH (melanocyte stimulating (hormone) which increases skin pigmentation. In man it remains rudimentary and is made up of colloid filled cysts or follicles. Cells secrete ACTH, MSH, endorphins and lipotrophins.

Between the pars intermedia and pars distalis are occasional fluid-filled cysts lined by cuboidal cells which are the only vestiges of the lumen of Rathke's pouch.

Pars tuberalis: This region is an extension of the glandular pituitary gland and its cells resemble those of the pars intermedia and pars distalis. The specific function of the cells in the pars tuberalis is not clear.

Microanatomy

Pars distalis: Clumps and cords of acidophils and basophils separated by strands of connective tissue along with capillaries engorged with blood are seen. In the acidophils granules in the cytoplasm stain red. The granules in the basophils are stained dark blue whereas the chromophobes lack granules so they have a pale blue cytoplasm.

Pars intermedia consists of cells which are highly basophilic and form irregular clumps between pars distalis and pars nervosa. It also contains a number of small cysts filled with eosinophilic material which represents the remains of the cavity of Rathke's pouch.

Pars nervosa contains cells called pituicytes and unmyelinated nerve fibers from the hypothalamic nuclei are seen. The hormones of neurohypophysis are stored in the expanded nerve terminals of nerve fibers called **Herring bodies** which appear as small islands of eosin stained substance. Pituicytes are modified glial cells as they are similar in structure and function (supportive) to the neuroglial cells of central nervous system. Only oval nuclei are seen not the scanty cytoplasm.

- The middle layer is zona fasciculata in which polyhedral cells are arranged radially in straight cords, one/two cells thick separated by fenestrated sinusoidal capillaries. The nucleus is vesicular light and centrally located and cytoplasm stains lightly and is often "foamy" in appearance (due to lipid droplets).
- Deep to this is zona reticularis consisting of irregular network of branching cords of small cells with a large nucleus containing only a small amount of lipid so cytoplasm stains pink with eosin separated by irregularly arranged sinusoidal space (fenestrated).
- The adrenal medulla is composed of closely packed clusters of **secretory cells** (pheochromocytes) supported by collagen fibers containing numerous wide diameter capillaries and veins. The secretory cells are basophilic with a large nucleus. They are called chromaffin cells because granules can be stained with chromium salts (potassium dichromate) which oxidizes catecholamines to a brown pigment by a process called chromaffin reaction. A few sympathetic ganglion cells are also present.

Keys for identification: Adrenal gland

a. Capsule is outermost.
b. Cortex consists of 3 zones—zona glomerulosa, zona fasciculata and zona reticularis.
c. Medulla consists of pheochromocytes, sympathetic ganglion cells and large capillaries.

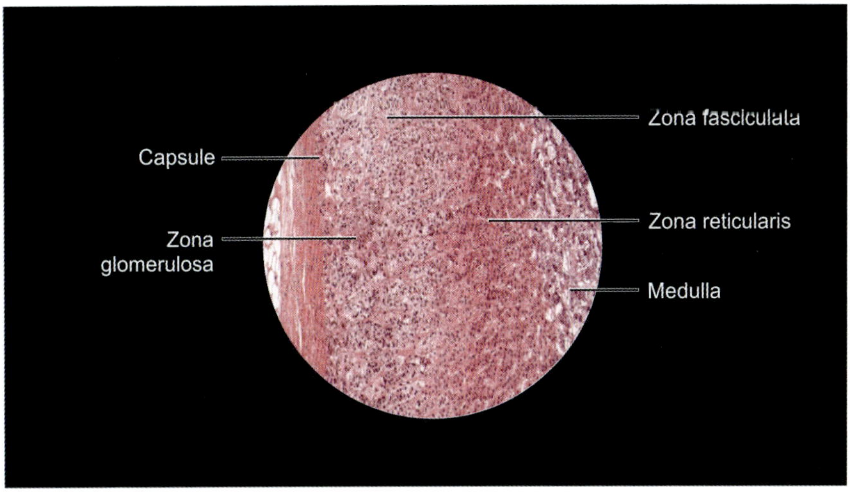

Fig. 3.55 Adrenal gland

Blank space for sketch work by students

PANCREAS (FIG. 3.56)

The pancreas is both an endocrine as well as an exocrine gland. Endocrine part forms 1-2% of total volume of the organ. There are about 1-2 millions islet of Langerhans (maximum) in the tail of pancreas). The pancreas produces the hormones insulin, glucagon and somatostatin directly into the bloodstream, which is termed an endocrine function. Insulin stimulates the synthesis of glycogen, protein and fatty acids. It also facilitates the uptake of glucose into cells and activates glucokinase in liver cells. The alpha cells which are at the periphery are 20% and they produce glucagon. Five percent are delta-cells which secrete somatostatin, a locally acting hormone which inhibits other endocrine cells. Activity of the two major islet cells alpha and beta is regulated by blood glucose levels. Increase in the blood glucose level stimulates beta cells to release insulin and inhibits alpha cells from releasing glucagon.

Microanatomy

The pancreas is surrounded by a very thin connective tissue capsule that invaginates into the gland to form septae, which divides it into lobules.

The light staining cells are the **pancreatic islets**. Each islet is an egg shaped mass 100-200 micrometers in diameter consisting up to 3000 secretory cells between which lie the blood capillaries surrounded by pericapillary space into which hormones are delivered first. Beta-cells are more than 60% located centrally in the islet and secrete insulin.

Keys for identification: Pancreas

a. Serous acini with centroacinar cells seen.
b. Presence of islet of Langerhans.
c. Absence of striated ducts.

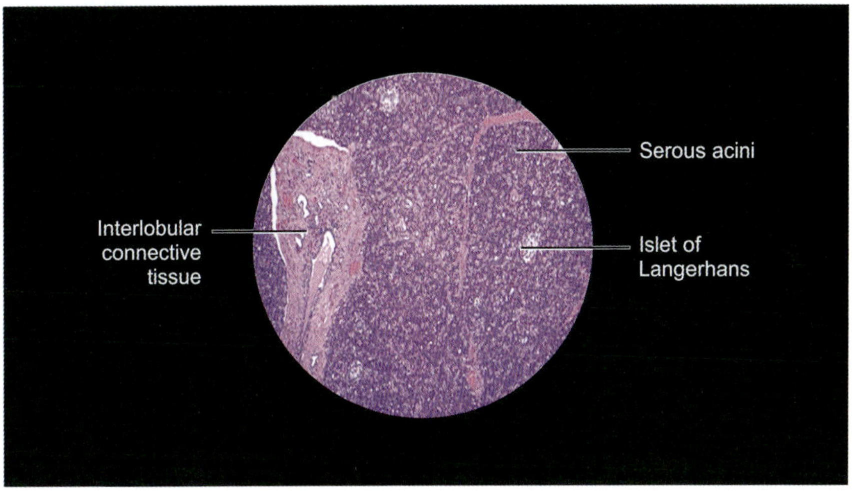

Fig. 3.56 Pancreas

Blank space for sketch work by students

PINEAL GLAND (FIG. 3.57)

It is a small organ connected to the brain by nerve fibers. It secretes melatonin which regulates the circadian rhythm of the body, effects on ageing and regulation of immune system.

Microanatomy

- The pineal gland is surrounded by a very thin **capsule** formed by **pia mater** which sends trabeculae into the gland forming lobules.
- Two types of cells are seen, **parenchymal and glial cells** along with **brain sand**.
- Parenchyma consists of **pinealocytes** (develop from neuroectodermal cells). They are highly modified neurons arranged in clusters and cords surrounded by numerous fenestrated capillaries. They have pale staining rounded nuclei with prominent nucleoli, granular cytoplasm and a large number of branched processes. The cytoplasmic granules contain melatonin and its precursor serotonin.
- Neuroglial cells resembling the **astrocytes** are seen between pinealocytes and associated with the capillaries. The nuclei of the glial cells are small and darkly stained.
- As age advances concentric layers of calcium and magnesium phosphate in an organic matrix are seen. They are called brain sand or **corpora arenacea**.

Keys for identification: Pineal gland

a. Pinealocytes with pale staining cytoplasm seen.
b. Darkly stained neuroglial cells are present.
c. Brain sand may be seen.

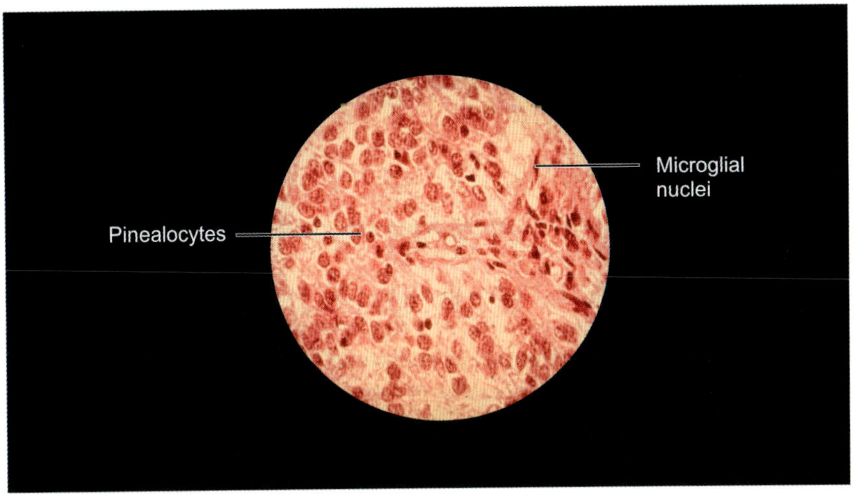

Fig. 3.57 Pineal gland

Blank space for sketch work by students

NERVOUS SYSTEM

The central nervous system (CNS) includes cerebrum, cerebellum and spinal cord.

CEREBRUM (CORTEX) (FIG. 3.58)

The cortex consists of outer gray matter and inner white matter.
- Inner most gray masses are known as basal ganglia.
- Gray matter is known as cortex and is 1.5–4.5 mm in thickness; convoluted in man, smooth in lower animals.

Microanatomy

- Cortex exhibits six layers:
  1. *Outermost molecular layer*—contains few cells, more fibers which run parallel to the surface.
  2. *Outer granular nerve cells* (8–10 mm in diameter).
  3. *Pyramidal cell layer*—contains small and medium sized, pyramidal shaped neurons.
  4. *Inner granular layer*—contains mainly stellate or granule cells.
  5. *Ganglionic or internal pyramidal cell layer*—contains big cells. In motor cortex, they are the largest and are known as 'Betz cells'.
  6. *Polymorphous cell layer*—because the cells in this layer have different shapes.
- Sections through different parts of the cortex show same general plan with some differences by which the site of the section is identified.
- *Neuroglia* are present in all the layers.
- About 10 billion **neurons** are present in the cerebral cortex and because one neuron can establish synaptic connections with as many as 1,00,000 others, the possibilities with regard to the number of available pathways are over whelming.
- White matter contains interlacing bundles of myelinated nerve fibers, having no neurilemma sheath.
- *In hematoxylin and eosin stain.* Cerebrum shows pale color, almost structureless appearing background—known as neuropil and consists of framework of naked nerve fibers and processes of neuroglia cells.
- Dark round nuclei of oligodendrocytes lie close to the white matter.
- Nucleoli of astrocytes are not prominent as those of neurons.
- *Motor and premotor areas are characterized by agranular* (absence of granules) cortex while **sensory areas are characterized by granular cortex**.

Keys for identification: Cerebrum (cortex)

a. Molecular layer.
b External granular layer.
c Pyramidal cell layer.
d. Internal granular layer.
e. Ganglionic layer.
f. Multiform layer.
g. Third and fifth layers are characteristic and contain pyramidal cells.

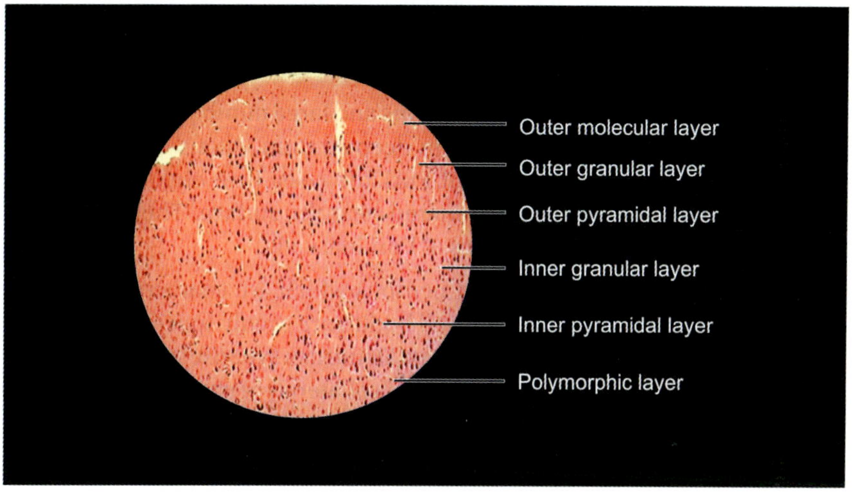

Fig. 3.58 Cerebral cortex

Blank space for sketch work by students

CEREBELLUM (FIG. 3.59)

- Cerebellum serves to coordinate the voluntary movements and maintain the normal posture and equilibrium.
- It consists of **outer gray matter and inner core of white matter**.
- Deep inside the white matter lie four pairs of cerebellar nuclei.
- Grossly cortex shows folds called folia.

Microanatomy

- **Cortex** shows three layers.
- **Outermost** is molecular layer, it stains light with eosin.
- **Middle** is purkinje cell layer.
- **Inner layer** is granular which stains intensely with hematoxylin.

Molecular layer: It contains relatively few neurons and large numbers of unmyelinated fibers. It shows small stellate cells and basket cells in deep stratum. Axons of the basket cells form baskets (network) around the cell bodies of Purkinje cells. One basket cells synapses with seventy Purkinje cells. Stellate cells are scattered near the surface. There dendrites synapse with parallel fibers and axons with dendrites of Purkinje cells.

Purkinje cells: Are large, flat, flask-shaped neurons which are characteristic of cerebellum. A single row of Purkinje cells is present and cell bodies are evenly spaced. The dendrites show arborization in molecular layer and bear spines. Dendrites synapse with parallel fibers, axon of stellate cells, climbing olivocerebellar fibers and collaterals of basket cells. The axons are the only efferents which passes through granular layer and end in nuclei of cerebellum.

Inner granular layer: Darkly stained, contains numerous, round granule cells of Golgi type II with large nuclei. The spaces not occupied by these cells are called **cerebellar islands**. These islands are occupied by glomeruli. Axons of granule cells branch in the form of "T", so that the axons make contact with the dendrites of Purkinje and basket cells. Glomeruli are seen in this layer, formed by dendrites of granule cells and axons of Golgi cells, synapsing with terminals of mossy fibers. Brush cells are also seen in the granular layer which are monodendritic.

All the intrinsic neurons of cerebellar cortex are inhibitiory except granule cells which are excitatory.

White matter: Contains central core of myelinated nerve fibers.
Two types of afferent fibers are seen in cerebellum.

1. **Climbing fibers** which pass through granular layer and reach the Purkinje cells dendrites in molecular layer.
2. **Mossy fibers** are other white fibers which synapse in granular layer.

Keys for identification: Cerebellum

a. Outer molecular layer.
b. Middle Purkinje cell layer.
c. Inner granular layer.

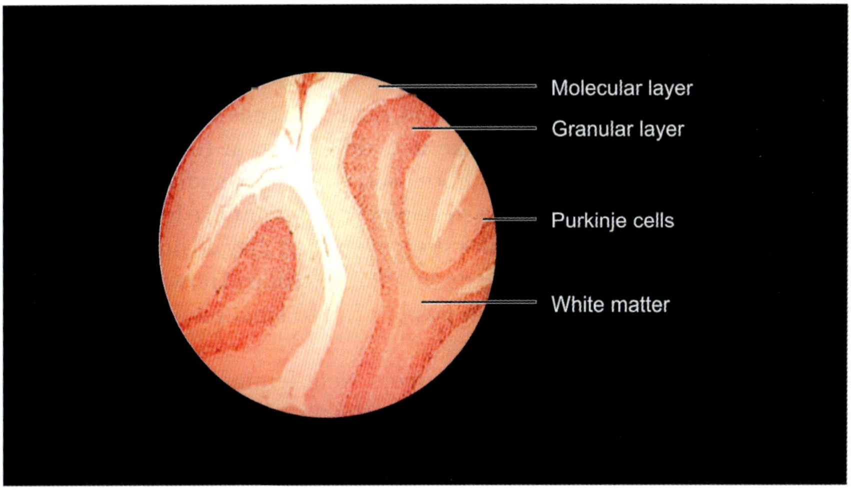

Fig. 3.59 Cerebellum

Blank space for sketch work by students

SPINAL CORD (FIGS 3.60 AND 3.61)

- Ovoid in transverse section. Contains inner gray matter and outer white matter unlike cerebellum.
- Gray matter is in the form of right and left columns connected with each other in the middle giving the appearance of letter 'H' in TS.
- Anterior horns are broader and shorter and do not reach the surface of the spinal cord. Posterior horns are thinner, longer and reach surface of the spinal cord.
- Lateral horns are present in thoracic and upper two lumbar segments and their cells are connected with sympathetic fibers.
- Gray matter contains nerve cells, nerve fibers, neuroglia cells and blood vessels.
- Neuroglia are arranged in a sponge-like network except at two places where they are condensed, one at the tips of posterior horns and other surrounding the central canal.
- Nerve cells are multipolar and vary in size. Golgi type-I cells have long axons which pass to the white matter. Golgi type-II cells have short axons and they do not leave the gray matter.
- Cell bodies of multipolar neurons are distributed in groups known as nuclei. Cell bodies in anterior horns are the largest and in posterior horn smallest whereas in lateral horns, intermediate in size.
- White matter consists of myelinated nerve fibers. Neurilemma sheath is absent and are cut transversely. In TS spinal cord is surrounded by the three meninges.

Keys for identification: Spinal cord

a. Outer white matter.
b. Inner H-shaped gray matter.
c. Central canal is present.

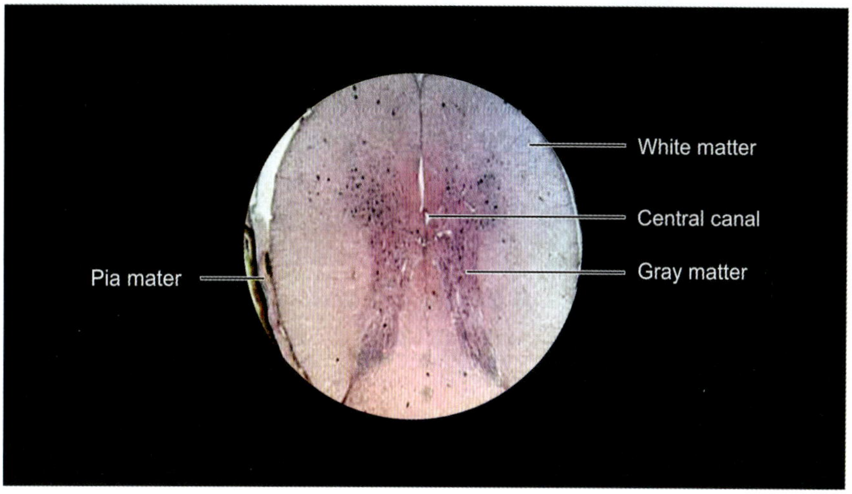

Fig. 3.60 Spinal cord

Blank space for sketch work by students

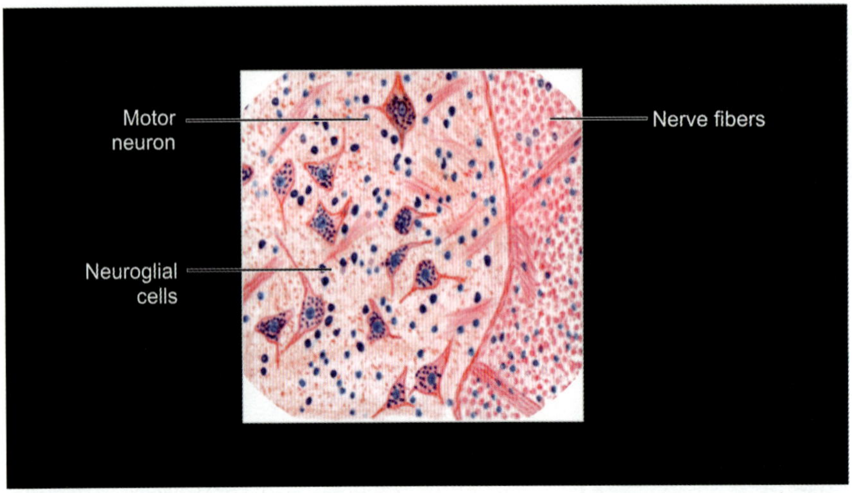

Fig. 3.61 Gray and white matter of spinal cord

Blank space for sketch work by students

EYE

- Eye is highly specialized sensory organ for sight.
- It consists of eyeball and accessory structures like conjunctiva, eyelids and lacrimal gland.
- There are three concentric coats of eyeball which enclose three chambers namely, anterior, posterior and vitreous.
- From within outwards three coats are:
  1. *Retina*—photosensitive layer.
  2. Middle vascular layer of **choroid in posterior 5/6th, ciliary body and iris in anterior 1/6th**.
  3. Outer most coat of **sclera in posterior 5/6th** and **cornea in anterior 1/6th**.

RETINA (FIG. 3.62)

The inner most lining of photosensitive layer is retina. It is transparent, soft and pinkish in color due to visual purple or rhodopsin, light bleaches retina. It cosists of ten layers, from without inwards they are as follows:

1. *Pigment layer*—formed by cuboidal, pigmented cells, attached firmly to **Bruch's** membrane of choroid and contains fuscin pigment.

   Apical part projects between rods and cones and are joined to these photoreceptors which explains the retinal detachment at these sites.

   The pigment absorbs light after photoreceptors are stimulated which creates a dark chamber effect in the eye and prevents reflection of light.

   Main functions of pigment layer:
   a. Absorption of light.
   b. Phagocytose tips of rods by lysosomes in them.
   c. Structural and metabolic support for rods and cones.
   d. Storage, esterification and release of vitamin A by smooth endoplasmic reticulum of basal region.
2. *Layer of rods and cones*—are dendrites of photoreceptor cells. Rods are more numerous than cones, except at macula lutea where only cones are present.
3. *External limiting membrane*—is a series of junctional complexes between apices of **Muller** cells and photoreceptors.
4. *Outer nuclear layer*—formed by cell bodies of rods and cones.
5. *Outer plexiform layer*—formed by cell bodies of bipolar neurons, horizontal cells, amacrine cells. Blood vessels from inner part of retina extend as far as this layer.
6. *Inner nuclear layer*—formed by cell bodies of bipolar neurons, horizontal cells, amacrine cells. Blood vessels from inner part of retina extend as far as this layer.
7. *Inner plexiform layer*—formed by synapses between axons of bipolar cells and dendrites of ganglionic cells and processes of amacrine cells.
8. *Ganglionic cell layer*—consists of large multipolar neurons with euchromatic nuclei and neuroglial cells. At macula lutea ganglion cells are arranged in single row. They receive input from bipolar cells and their axons form optic nerve.
9. *Layer of nerve fibers*—called **stratum opticum**. Bundles of unmyelinated axons of ganglionic cells converge towards the optic disc and passes through lamina cribrosa to form optic

nerve. There is neither myelin sheath nor sheath of Schwann cells. Outside the eyeball they are myelinated by oligodendrocytes.

10. *Inner limiting membrane*—homogeneous delicate layer formed by expanded bases of Muller cells and basement membrane.

Keys for identification: Retina

a. Outermost pigment cell layer.
b. Middle plexiform and nuclear layer.
c. Innermost internal limiting membrane.

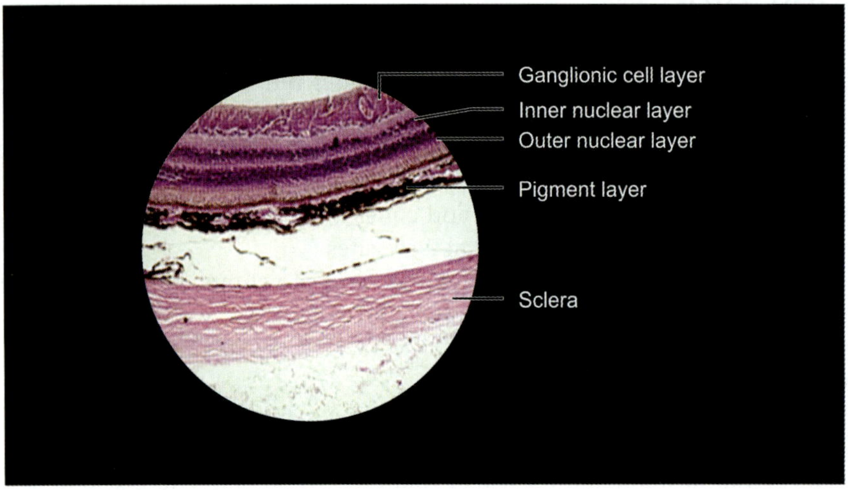

Fig. 3.62 Retina

Blank space for sketch work by students

CORNEA (FIG. 3.63)

- Cornea is colorless, transparent, anterior one-fifth of the outer coat and continues behind with sclera at limbus.
- It is avascular and nutrition is by diffusion through aqueous humour of anterior chamber.
- It has greater refractive index than lens.
- It is thicker in the center (0.7 mm) than periphery (1.1 mm).
- It consists of five layers.
  1. *Corneal epithelium:* Made of stratified squamous nonkeratinized epithelium (5–6 layers) and no papillae.
     - It has rich nerve supply and remarkable regenerative capacity.
     - It is continuous with conjunctiva at limbus.
  2. *Bowman's membrane:* (10–12 microns)
     - It is homogeneous acellular layer beneath the corneal epithelium.
     - It is the condensation of connective tissue lamina propria which is a protective layer and provides stability and strength to cornea.
  3. *Substantia propria:* It constitutes 90% of the corneal tissue.
     - It is fibrous, tough, unyielding and transparent.
     - It is composed of 60 lamellae of collagen fibrils arranged in an orderly manner, parallel to surface cornea.
     - These fibrils are bound together by hyaluronic acid and chondroitin sulphate.
     - In between stellate shaped spaces are present corneal corpuscles.
  4. *Descemet's membrane:* Homogeneous acellular layer made of membrane.
     - It breaks to form trabecular tissue on inner wall of sclera.
     - Spaces between the trabeculae (Fontana) communicate with anterior chamber and canal of Schlemm.
  5. *Mesothelium/Endothelium:* A single layer of flat polygonal cells, squamous or cuboidal cover the posterior surface of cornea and is reflected on the front of iris.

Keys for identification: Cornea

a. Outer most layer is nonkeratinized stratified squamous epithelium.
b. In between anterior and posterior limiting membranes there is a layer of substantia propria which contains several layers of collagen fibers.
c. Innermost layer is lined by single layer of cuboidal or flat cells.

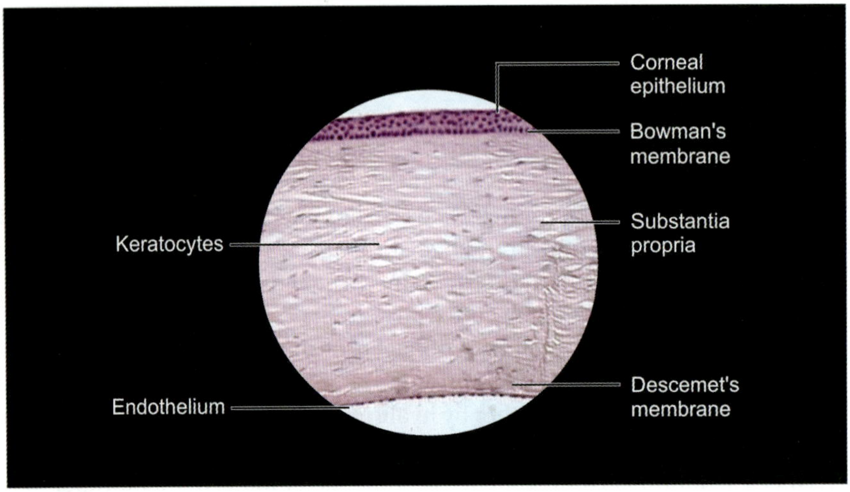

Fig. 3.63 Cornea

Blank space for sketch work by students

EYELIDS (FIG. 3.64)

- The two movable folds of skin in front of eye are called eyelids.
- They protect the eye from injury and excessive light.
- From without inwards it consists of following:
  1. Skin is the outer lining. Dermis contains sebaceous and sweat glands.
  2. Subcutaneous tissue of loose areolar type and devoid of fat.
  3. Muscle layer—striated muscle, orbicularis oculi, palpebral part is present. It is parallel to palpebral fissure.
  4. Loose areolar tissue—contains blood vessels and nerves and continuous with aponeurotic layer of scalp.
  5. Tarsal plate—dense fibrous tissue.
  6. Tarsal glands are modified sebaceous glands (Meibomian glands) which lie between tarsi and conjunctiva. They open at free margins of eyelids.
  7. Conjunctiva-palpebral conjunctiva is transparent mucous membrane lining the inner surface of eyelids and reflected on eyeball over sclera and cornea. It has stratified columnar cells (2–3 layers) and goblet cells. The ocular conjunctiva is stratified squamous epithelium.

Keys for identification: Eyelid

a. Outer layer is lined by keratinized stratified squamous epithelium.
b. Dermis contains sebaceous (glands of Zeis), sweat glands (glands of Moll) and hair follicle. It is devoid of fat.
c. There is dense fibroelastic plate next to skin.
d. The skeletal muscle layer (orbicularis oculi) lies superficial to tarsal plate.
e. Within the tarsal plate lies vertically oriented Meibomian glands.

39. *Palatine Tonsil*
    a. Aggregations of lymphatic tissue forming lymphatic nodules and germinal center.
    b. It is covered by stratified squamous nonkeratinized epithelium.
    c. The epithelium invaginates to form tonsillar crypts.

40. *Lungs*
    a. Numerous thin walled hollow spaces (Honeycomb appearance of alveoli) seen.
    b. Lining epithelium of alveoli is simple squamous type.
    c. Intrapulmonary bronchi, bronchioles and respiratory bronchioles are seen.

41. *Epiglottis*
    a. Elastic cartilage in the middle.
    b. Stratified squamous epithelium on one side.
    c. Pseudostratified ciliated columnar epithelium on the other side.

42. *Trachea*
    a. Epithelium lined by pseudostratified columnar ciliated epithelium.
    b. Serous and mucous acini present.
    c. C shaped hyaline cartilage seen.

43. *Elastic Artery (Large Artery)*
    a. Tunica intima lined by endothelial cells (simple squamous epithelium).
    b. Tunica media rich in elastic fibers and few smooth muscle fibers.
    c. Tunica adventitia consists of areolar tissue and has vasa vasorum.

44. *Muscular Artery (Medium Size Artery)*
    a. Tunica intima is lined by endothelial cells.
    b. Tunica media is well separated from intima by prominent internal elastic lamina.
    c. Tunica media is composed mainly of circular smooth muscle fibers.
    d. Vasa vasorum is absent in tunica adventitia.

45. *Large Vein*
    a. Wall is thin and lumen is collapsed and larger than artery.
    b. Absence of internal elastic lamina.
    c. Tunica media is thin with circular smooth muscle fiber.
    d. Thickest coat is tunica adventitia with longitudinal smooth muscles and vasa vasorum.

46. *Submandibular Salivary Gland*
    a. Both serous and mucous acini but predominantly serous.
    b. Serous crescents (demilunes of Giannuzzi) are the characteristic feature.
    c. Number of ducts are few.

47. *Parotid Salivary Gland*
    a. Serous acini with narrow lumen.
    b. Number of ducts are more.
    c. Centrally placed round nuclei in the serous acini.

48. *Sublingual Gland*
    a. Mucous acini with a large lumen.
    b. Flat nucleus placed near the base of the mucous cells.
    c. Very few ducts are present.

49. *Thin Skin (Hairy Skin)*
   a. Thin epidermis of nonkeratinized stratified squamous epithelium.
   b. Dermis contains hair follicles and sebaceous glands.
   c. Arrector pilorum muscle.

50. *Thick Skin (Glabrous Skin)*
   a. No hair follicles.
   b. Thick epidermis of keratinized stratified squamous epithelium.
   c. Prominent dermal and epidermal papillae.

51. *Tongue*
   a. Nonkeratinized stratified squamous epithelium.
   b. Presence of papillae.
   c. Inner layer contains skeletal muscles and glands.

52. *Circumvallate Papilla*
   a. Nonkeratinized stratified squamous epithelium.
   b. Numerous taste buds in the groove.
   c. Presence of serous glands of von Ebner.

53. *Filiform Papilla*
   a. Keratinized stratified squamous epithelium.
   b. Finger-shaped projections.
   c. Skeletal muscles seen in it.

54. *Fungiform Papilla*
   a. Nonkeratinized stratified squamous epithelium.
   b. Mushroom-shaped structure.
   c. Skeletal muscle seen inside.

55. *Esophagus (TS)*
   a. Nonkeratinized stratified squamous epithelium.
   b. Submucosa contains glands.
   c. Muscularis mucosa is prominent.
   d. Muscularis externa containing inner circular and outer longitudinal smooth muscle layer.

56. *Stomach (Fundus) TS*
   a. Simple columnar epithelium.
   b. Straight tube like glands with gastric pits shorter and glands larger.
   c. Glands present red stained oxyntic cells and blue stained peptic cells in lamina propria.
   d. Muscularis externa containing inner oblique, middle circular and outer longitudinal smooth muscle layer.

57. *Stomach (Pyloric Part) TS*
   a. Simple columnar epithelium.
   b. Mucous secreting glands shorter and gastric pits larger and deep.
   c. Thickest middle circular muscle layer forming pyloric sphincter.

58. *Duodenum (TS)*
    a. Brunner's glands in submucosa.
    b. Few goblet cells in mucous membrane.
    c. Simple columnar epithelium with numerous villi.
    d. Crypts of Lieberkuhn present.

59. *Jejunum (TS)*
    a. Simple columnar epithelium with tall villi with goblet cells.
    b. Absence of Brunner's glands in submucosa.
    c. Absence of peyer's patches.

60. *Ileum (TS)*
    a. Simple columnar epithelium with small villi.
    b. Crypts of Lieberkuhn present.
    c. Mucosa containing Peyer's patches.

61. *Large Intestine (Colon) (TS)*
    a. Simple columnar epithelium.
    b. Numerous goblet cells.
    c. Mucosa with folds but absence of villi.
    d. Prominent *Taenia coli.*

62. *Appendix (TS)*
    a. Thicker muscular wall.
    b. Presence of lumen but no folds (villi are absent).
    c. Intestinal glands few in number.
    d. Lymphatic nodules in submucosa (lamina propria).
    e. Simple columnar epithelium.

63. *Liver*
    a. Numbers of liver (hepatic) lobules (hexagonal areas).
    b. Central vein with radiating sinusoids (empty spaces) and liver (hepatic) cells.
    c. At the periphery of lobule, portal triad (branch of portal vein, hepatic artery and bile duct present).

64. *Gallbladder*
    a. Simple columnar epithelium with brush border.
    b. Dancing mucous membrane.
    c. No muscularis mucosa and no goblet cells.
    d. Serous or fibrous coat.

65. *Pancreas*
    a. Main bulk contains darkly stained numerous serous acini having basophilic bases and eosinophilic apical part.
    b. Presence of lightly stained islets of Langerhans—Rounded bodies arranged in small clumps and scattered in between the acini.

66. *Kidney*
   a. Renal corpuscles (glomerulus), proximal and distal convoluted tublues in cortex.
   b. Renal tubules (Henle's loop and collecting ducts) in medulla.

67. *Ureter (TS)*
   a. Small star shaped lumen with smooth and regular folds.
   b. Mucous membrane lined by transitional epithelium.
   c. Outer circular and inner longitudinal muscle coat.

68. *Urinary Bladder (TS)*
   a. Mucous membrane lined by transitional epithelium.
   b. Thick muscle coat. Inner and outer longitudinal and middle circular muscle coat.
   c. External surface is serous coat.

69. *Urethra*
   a Mucosa is lined by transitional or pseudostratified columnar or stratified columnar or stratified squamous epithelium.
   b. Lumen is irregular.
   c. Irregular venous spaces surround the lumen.

70. *Testis*
   a. Number of seminiferous tubules of various shapes and size.
   b. Seminiferous epithelium containing spermatozoa of various stages.
   c. Lumen may contain sperms.
   d. In between tubules, presence of blood vessels, connective tissue and interstitial cells of Leydig.

71. *Epididymis (TS)*
   a. Consists of long convoluted ducts cut at various places.
   b. Lined by ciliated pseudostratified columnar epithelium.
   c. Clumps of sperm within lumen.

72. *Vas Deferens (TS)*
   a. Wall is very thick and lumen very small and stellate.
   b. Outer fibrous coat.
   c. Thick middle muscular coat.
   d. Lined by ciliated pseudostratified tall columnar epithelium.
   e. Lumen may contain sperms.

73. *Seminal Vesicle*
   a. Lined by pseudostratified epithelium.
   b. Mucous membrane presents numerous branching and anastomosis, giving honeycomb appearance.
   c. Muscular coat of inner circular muscle and outer longitudinal muscle.

74. *Prostate*
   a. Fibromuscular capsule and stroma.
   b. Number of follicles with wide lumen and irregular lumen.
   c. Follicles may contain amyloid body (corpora amylacea).
   d. Prostratic acini lined by simple columnar epithelium.

75. *Penis*
  a. Outer covering of skin.
  b. Three masses of erectile tissues.
  c. Centrally placed artery in each corpus cavernosus.
  d. Two dorsal arteries and vein on dorsal aspect.

76. *Ovary*
  a. Surface—Tunica albuginea with cuboidal germinal epithelium.
  b. Outer cortex contains ovarian follicles of various size and maturity.
  c. Inner medulla contains connective tissue and blood vessels.

77. *Uterine Tube (Fallopian Tube) (TS)*
  a. Mucous membrane lined by ciliated columnar epithelium.
  b. Mucous membrane shows numerous branching and folding.
  c. Outer longitudinal and inner circular muscle coats.

78. *Uterus (Proliferative Phase)*
  a. Very thick muscle layer.
  b. Mucous membrane (endometrium) lined by simple columnar epithelium.
  c. Myometrium is thick with numerous blood vessels.
  d. Lamina propria containing simple tubular uterine glands. 'Straight glands' in proliferative phase.

79. *Uterus (Secretory Phase)*
  a. Myometrium with numerous blood vessels.
  b. Thick mucous membrane (thick endometrium) lined by simple columnar epithelium.
  c. Lamina propria containing simple tubular uterine glands. 'Coiled or tortuous glands' in secretory phase.

80. *Vagina*
  a. Lined by stratified squamous nonkeratinized epithelium.
  b. No glands.
  c. Numerous elastic fibers present in adventitia.

81. *Mammary Gland (Resting Stage)*
  a. Lobules of glandular tissue.
  b. Ducts predominate and few acini or acinar lobules.
  c. Abundant fibrofatty tissue separating the lobules.

82. *Mammary Gland (Active or Lactating Stage)*
  a. Lobules contain more prominent acini, lined by cuboidal epithelium.
  b. Connective tissue separating the lobules or duct system is scanty or minimal.

83. *Placenta*
  a. The villi are lined by an epithelium having an inner layer of cytotrophoblast and outer layer of syncytiotrophoblast.
  b. These villi contain fetal capillaries with nucleated RBCs and fetal connective tissue in the core of the villus.
  c. Maternal blood is present in the intervillous space.

84. *Umbilical Cord*
   a. Two umbilical arteries.
   b. One umbilical vein.
   c. Wharton's jelly (mucoid tissue) is present.

85. *Pituitary Gland (Hypophysis Cerebri)*
   a. Pars anterior cellular (rich in cells and sinusoids) and some acidophil and basophil cells are found.
   b. Pars intermedia—thin sheets of blue staining cells.
   c. Pars nervosa—consists of light stained nerve fibers and pituicytes.

86. *Thyroid Gland*
   a. Number of thyroid follicles containing pink stained eosinophilic colloid and lined by cuboidal epithelium.
   b. Small amount of intercellular connective tissue and parafollicular cells.

87. *Parathyroid Gland*
   a. Lightly stained masses of cells. Most of these are chief cells (only nuclei are seen and oxyphil cells (large eosinophilic cells with pink cytoplasm).
   b. Good amount of blood capillaries.

88. *Suprarenal Gland (Adrenal Gland)*
   a. Covered by capsule with trabeculae.
   b. Cortex consists of zona glomerulosa, zona fasciculata and zona reticularis.
   c. Zona glomerulosa—cells arranged in inverted V shaped manner.
   d. Zona fasciculata—cells arranged in fascicles or straight columns.
   e. Zona reticularis—cord of cells forming network.
   f. Medulla showing sinusoids and sympathetic ganglion cells.
   g. Groups of cells (basophilic) separated by wide sinusoids.

89. *Pineal Gland*
   a. Pinealocytes with pale staining cytoplasm seen.
   b. Darkly stained neuroglial cells are present.
   c. Brain sand may be seen.

90. *Cornea*
   a. Outer most layer is nonkeratinized stratified squamous epithelium.
   b. In between anterior and posterior limiting membrances there is a layer of substantia propria which contains several layers of collagen fibers.
   c. Innermost layer is lined by single layer of cuboidal or flat cells.

91. *Retina*
   a. Outermost pigment cell layer.
   b. Middle plexiform and nuclear layer.
   c. Innermost internal limiting membrane.

92. *Eyelid*
    a. Outer layer is lined by keratinized stratified squamous epithelium.
    b. Dermis contains sebaceous (glands of Zeis), sweat glands (glands of Moll) and hair follicle. It is devoid of fat.
    c. There is dense fibroelastic plate next to skin.
    d. The skeletal muscle layer (orbicularis oculi) lies superficial to tarsal plate.
    e. Within the tarsal plate lies vertically oriented meibomian glands.

93. *Lacrimal Gland*
    a. Compound tubuloalveolar serous gland.
    b. Secretory unit is surrounded by myoepithelial cells inside the basement membrane.
    c. Fatty droplets are seen in the cell.
    d. Lacrimal gland is differentiated from parotid and pancreas by the lumen of acinus which is largest in lacrimal gland and smallest in pancreas and intralobular ducts are prominent in lacrimal gland.

94. *Cerebrum (Cortex)*
    a. Molecular layer.
    b. External granular layer.
    c. Pyramidal cell layer.
    d. Internal granular layer.
    e. Ganglionic layer.
    f. Multiformic layer.
    g. 3rd and 5th layers are characteristic and contain pyramidal cells.

95. *Cerebellum*
    a. Outer molecular layer.
    b. Middle Purkinje cell layer.
    c. Inner granular layer.

96. *Spinal Cord*
    a. Outer white matter.
    b. Inner H-shaped gray matter.
    c. Central canal is present.

Index

Page numbers followed by *f* refer to figure

D

E

F

G

N

O

P

T

U

V

W

Z